# Childhood Marital Conflict, Adult Anger

Israel Dibbert

**Abstract**

The study sought to examine the relationship between witnessing verbal marital conflict as a child and behavioral anger responses in adulthood. An underlying premise for the study was that verbal marital conflict could be an underlying cause of developmental and behavioral problems in adults who witnessed verbal marital conflict as a child. Previous studies focused on marital conflict in regards to physical conflict, leaving out verbal conflict. One hundred participants, who acknowledged witnessing verbal marital conflict as children, completed the Novaco Anger Scale (NAS; Novaco, 1994, 2003) and the Children's Perception of Interparental Conflict Scale (CPIC; Grych et al., 1992). Participants showed average anger responses and sometimes low anger responses, which did not show significant correlation with exposure to parental verbal marital conflict as children. The findings provided implications for future research which included conducting another study with the same research question, but using a qualitative approach to provide in-depth knowledge on exposure to verbal marital conflict as a child and behavioral anger responses in adulthood, while also using a quantitative approach to examine the behavioral effect. It further suggested identifying the need for person-centered intervention, and enhancing models of skill training for handling anger and relationships.

## Table of Contents

CHAPTER 1. INTRODUCTION .................................................................. 1

    Background of the Problem (Introduction) ............................................ 1

    Statement of the Problem ........................................................................ 8

    Purpose of the Study ............................................................................... 9

    Significance of the Study ...................................................................... 11

    Research Design .................................................................................... 13

    Research Questions and Hypotheses .................................................... 15

    Assumptions and Limitations ............................................................... 15

    Definition of Terms .............................................................................. 17

    Expected Findings ................................................................................ 19

    Organization of the Remainder of the Study ........................................ 20

CHAPTER 2. LITERATURE REVIEW ....................................................... 21

    Introduction to the Literature Review .................................................. 22

    Theoretical Orientation of the Study .................................................... 22

    Review of Research Literature and Methodological Literature ........... 30

    Summary to the Literature Review ....................................................... 51

CHAPTER 3. METHODOLOGY .................................................................. 53

    Purpose of the Study ............................................................................. 53

    Research Design .................................................................................... 53

    Target Population and Participant Selection ........................................ 55

| | |
|---|---|
| Procedures | 59 |
| Instruments | 62 |
| Research Questions and Hypotheses | 65 |
| Data Analysis | 66 |
| Ethical Considerations | 67 |
| Expected Findings | 69 |
| Summary | 70 |
| CHAPTER 4. DATA COLLECTION AND ANALYSIS | 71 |
| Introduction | 71 |
| Description of the Sample | 71 |
| Summary of the Results | 77 |
| Details of the Analysis and the Results | 79 |
| Conclusion | 84 |
| CHAPTER 5. DISCUSSION, IMPLICATIONS, RECOMMENDATIONS | 85 |
| Introduction | 85 |
| Summary of the Results | 85 |
| Discussion of the Results | 92 |
| Discussion of the Conclusions | 95 |
| Limitations | 100 |
| Recommendations for Future Research or Interventions | 103 |
| Conclusion | 107 |
| REFERENCES | 110 |

# CHAPTER 1. INTRODUCTION

## Introduction

Marriage presents an opportunity for families to raise their children in an environment that promotes social values and help the children create a good future. Sometimes the environment surrounding marriage could deny children the peace they require to foster appropriate growth. Marital conflict can be seen as a potential contributor to the development of future behavioral problems in children and adults (Cummings & Davies, 2011). The implication of marital conflict on children relates to the magnitude of the conflict and its escalation (Ablow, Measelle, Cowan, & Cowan, 2009). It further involves children witnessing the verbal and/or physical differences between their parents. This study assesses the correlation between witnessing verbal marital conflict as a child and behavioral anger responses in adulthood utilizing the theoretical framework of emotional security theory and social learning theory.

## Background of the Problem

Conflict is part of family life and marriage. Strong, DeVault, and Cohen (2011) explained the part of conflict in marriage stating that happy marriages are not free of conflict but have a positive role depending on how a couple handles conflicts. The difference between a happy marriage and a sad marriage is in the constructive or destructive nature in which the couple handles arising conflicts (Davies, Martin, & Ciccheti, 2012). Happy marriages will have positive strategies for handling any conflicts, while unhappy marriages will probably have ineffective strategies of dealing with conflicts. Regardless of how the couple handles their conflict, any disagreement occurring within the family has an impact on the children.

The difference in the impact will vary with children coming from homes where the couple is able to handle the conflict, in addition, being able to move beyond arising differences. For families where conflicts remain unresolved, the children could suffer in their academics, behavior, and emotional well-being (Cummings & Davies, 2011). The implication of marital conflict on a child is reflective of how the parents handle their affairs, and their recognition that their actions will affect their children with a high possibility of negative attribution. Continued conflicts and those with increased velocity of aggression are destructive to the well-being of a child (Ablow et al., 2009). However, finding a resolution means that the child is able to develop by identifying the challenges of a relationship and knowing it is possible to find amicable solutions.

Marital conflict has two extremes notably destructive and constructive (Strong et al., 2011). Each involves a range of behaviors (Cummings, Faircloth, Mitchell, Cummings, & Schermerhon, 2008). For example, destructive marital conflicts includes behaviors such as avoidance, inflexibility, escalating spirals including manipulation, threats and coercion, retaliation, competition, and insulting verbal and nonverbal behaviors such as criticizing, defensiveness, complaining, confrontation, and contempt of the other person. Constructive behaviors include adoption of communication traits such as clarification, and validating as well as support, affection, and problem solving as aspect of positive conflict. The focus of this research is the destructive element of conflict and its implications on child development. The expectation is that such conflicts affect the interactions of family members.

The family unit is an important part of the growth of a child as it provides the first place of socialization (Drisccoll & Nagel, 2011). In the family, children learn how to interact with others and model their interpersonal relationships that also inform future relationships including romantic ones (Bern, 2013). Having a positive environment at home encourages loving relationships building the character of the child to form healthy relationships in adulthood. Socialization within the family could however adopt a negative connotation when a child experiences abuse within the home (Drisccoll & Nagel, 2011). The receiver of the abuse may not be the child, but as an observer, the child will feel its impact on their development. Children brought up in abusive homes will expect the abuse to continue outside their home. Kindness will be a surprise to such a child compared to abuse.

Research shows that marital conflict has various implications on the life and development of children of conflicting parents (Davies et al., 2012; Fosco, DeBoard, & Grych, 2007; Laurent, Kim, & Capaldi, 2008; Pauli-Pott & Dieter, 2007; Sturge-Apple, Davies, Winter, Cummings, & Schermerhon, 2008). One effect is on the child's romantic relationships, where young adults coming from a background where their parents engaged in conflict had lower quality relationships because of the potential to engage in conflicts with their partners (Cui & Fincham, 2010). The indication of such findings is the possibility of intergenerational transmission of couple conflict.

According to Nicholas and Rasmussen (2006), parents could have a conflict without their children being aware. Example of an illustration, Jim and Jenny have a five-year-old son and a fourteen-year-old daughter. At breakfast, the children observe that although the mother is serving their father breakfast in the usual manner, her action seems somewhat restrained. In the evening, Jenny seems to be her jovial self. Her daughter asks her what was wrong that morning during breakfast. Jenny tells her daughter that sometimes people who love each other disagree, but their love can override the disagreement. She tells her daughter that love and family includes sometimes disagreeing, other times agreeing, and even agreeing to disagree. The lesson Jenny was teaching her daughter was that family and marriage were not perfect and could have disagreements. Nevertheless, this did not mean the children and other family members needed to feel the negative effect of the disagreement. Within such a family, the socialization of the children will revolve around knowing sometimes they could disagree with other people but they could find amicable solutions to such disagreements.

A contrasting family is when at breakfast the couple continues their argument in front of the children. An example of this illustration, John and Joy begin their argument in the privacy of their bedroom, but the children can hear the argument by the raised voices. The couple then takes the argument into the breakfast room, and leaves for work without having found a resolution. The argument could continue in the evening or the couple refuses to acknowledge each other. In such an environment, the children will realize their parents had a conflict and due to the lack of communication, one may not ask for details regarding the behavior. The children in this relationship may grow in fear of the fighting between their parents, an aspect that could also affect the emotional development of the children as well as other areas of their life (Fear et al., 2009).

Arising from the hypothetical illustrations provided is that marital conflict extends to the various levels of the family, affecting other persons that are not active in the conflict. Such persons become part of the conflict through emotional association (Nicholas & Rasmussen, 2006). For example, the daughter of Jenny became part of the disagreement by wanting to know what was happening between her parents. The mother, however, countered the possible negative implication by showing a constructive aspect in confrontations among children. The impact of marital conflict on children will be short-term and flow into the long-term, whether constructive or destructive. Continued exposure to destructive marital conflict causes children to develop maladaptive behavior compared to low exposure or witnessing positive inter-parental conflicts.

Children sometimes develop problem behaviors when exposed to couple's conflicts. Rhoades (2009) found that children exposed to conflict between their parents developed behavioral problems responding to the conflict. The literature shows two possible responses, namely avoidance and involvement behaviors (Keller, Cummings, Davies, & Lubje, 2007; Koss et al., 2012). Avoidance refers to children trying to stay away from their parental conflict; the avoidance is a conscious and active effort (Rhoades, 2009). Avoidance becomes evident through withdrawal and lack of resolution when faced with a conflict (Fisher, 2012; Sween, 2011; Thokala, 2009). Involvement denotes children trying to intervene in the conflict through physical interruption such as pulling on one parent when the argument is ongoing (Cummings & Davies, 2010). The child may also take the side of one parent if they actively become part of the conflict. Involvement and avoidance behaviors are an initial indicator in how children react to conflict and their future responses.

Exposure to parental conflict adds to the development of externalization and internalization behaviors in children (El-Sheikh et al., 2009; Fosco & Grych, 2008; Obradovic, Bush, & Boyce, 2011). The behaviors become evident through psychological challenges and achievement in the life of a child. For example, externalizing problems are visible in poor academic achievement for children coming from families with poor marital conflict resolution (Shelton & Haros, 2008). Behavioral outcomes signify the way parental conflict affects the life of a child. The behaviors adopted by children such as involvement or avoidance signify the internalization and externalization of the conflict. Children that are involved in the conflict could adopt behaviors relating to those of their parents such as becoming aggressive. A standard of behavior is not available that can define whether a child will want to become part of the conflict or avoid its triggers.

Continued exploration of internalization and externalization indicated that marital conflict affects children's psychological functioning especially through exposure to repeated instances of destructive conflict (El-Sheikh et al., 2013; Faircloth, 2012; Nigg et al., 2009; Zarling et al., 2013;). Depending on the degree of destructiveness, it can cause internalizing problems such as unhappiness and low self-esteem as well as externalizing behavioral problems such as criminal behavior, anger, decline in academic performance, social and interpersonal modification, and broad mental health encounters (El-Sheikh et al., 2013). Children exposed to constant marital conflicts suffer health related risks including emotional health. Considering the socialization of a child it becomes possible that following exposure, the child may not show negative effects.

Research shows a clear indication that children's exposure to marital conflict could lead to a negative effect on child development especially on emotional development as it causes fear, and anxiety (Davies & Cummings, 2010; Faircloth, 2012; Rhoades, 2009). Cases where the parents are able to resolve their conflicts promotes constructive behavior in children as they learn ways to address their problems. Constructive resolution of conflicts helps children develop problem solving skills.

Focus in research has been on the emotional aspect of exposure to couple conflict and especially on the future relationships of the child (Buehler & Welsh, 2009; Cummings, Kuoros, & Papp, 2007; Davies et al., 2012; Fosco & Grych, 2008; Richmond & Stocker, 2007). Researchers study whether a child that witnesses marital conflict will have a lower quality relationship such as an intimate relationship compared to children that do not witness such conflicts (Hare, Miga, & Allen, 2009; Lindahl & Malik, 2011; Hare, Miga, & Allen, 2009; Sturge-Apple et al., 2008). The agreement in literature is that children witnessing marital conflict will have poor quality relationships because of intergenerational impact. This means that the children as adults may tend to start confrontations with their partners and break up relationships.

The current research is grounded in emotional security theory (EST) and social learning theory (SLT) as the theoretical framework for this study. The research will add and expand EST by further understanding the relationship between verbal marital conflict as a child and behavioral anger responses as an adult measured by the Novaco Anger Scale (NAS; Novaco, 1994, 2003). Davies and Cummings (1994) developed EST in order to explain the coping and adaptation of psychological adjustment of children's reactions to interparental conflict. The theory speculates it is important to maintain emotional security in a child's life along with protection and safety as lack of emotional security poses problems for long-term functioning for children throughout their lives for example: academically, socially, and into adulthood (Davies & Cummings, 1994). Maintaining emotional security will aid a child in emotional experiences, action tendencies, and appraisal of self around family and socially (Davies, Winter & Cicchetti, 2006). EST also proposes that children's ability to cope and problem solve increases due to stress after witnessing interparental conflicts (Davies et al., 2006).

The use of SLT suggest that children who witness marital conflict quiet often will copy the disruptive and aggressive behavior of their parents which can result in the external behaviors inside and outside the home (Akers et al., 1979; Bandura, 1973). No research has been conducted to see if an adult who witnessed verbal marital conflict as a child will influence behavioral anger responses during adulthood measured by the Novaco Anger (NAS; Novaco, 1994, 2003); as such, this research will add to the existing theory SLT.

## Statement of the Problem

Research of the literature indicates that marital conflict negatively influences child development on an emotional level leading to development of internalization and externalization behaviors (Davies et al., 2006). Such behaviors signify the reaction of the child to witnessing conflicts. Much focus in research has been on marital conflict in general and especially on the response of children, and reaching the age of early adolescence. This leaves out the continued manifestation of witnessing marital conflict as a person matures into adulthood and beyond. The question left unanswered is whether witnessing marital conflict has a bearing on the behavior of a person as an adult. Noted in literature is that socialization, such as within the family unit, can explain why a person acts as they do showing it is an attribute of their background (Hersh, 2008). Children may not seem to be active participants in the conflict; however, they are active in the sense of observation and feelings associated with the conflict.

The literature available adequately portrays the impact of marital conflict, but does not show that of verbal marital conflict. This study seeks to respond to the aspect of verbal marital conflict identifying its impact on children and their behavior in childhood. Verbal marital conflict is a specific type of aggression, in which people fight via words (Cummings, 1998). It provides an opportunity for people to be abusive, and demeaning to their partners. Such behavior has a bearing on the psychological well-being of children as it can teach them to value or disvalue one or both of their parents (Sturge-Apple, Skibi, & Davies, 2012). For example, the child could undermine the abused parents considering them as inconsequential as they heard the dominant parent referring to their partner as such. The study looks at whether witnessing verbal marital conflict in childhood will impact how a person responds to anger in adulthood.

## Purpose of the Study

The purpose of this study is to explore the relationship between adult behavioral responses of anger and verbal marital conflict witnessed as a child. Current research studies on anger shows that children's first experience with anger is through their parents, where they could see parents arguing, and from this the children develop models of anger and conflict resolution (DeBaryshe & Fryxell, 2013). Children's interaction with their parents promote parental socialization from which children form a basis for their emotional development. Parent emotional socialization of their children occur through modeling, imitation, and exposure to various stimuli (Hersh, 2008). The emotional climate to which a child becomes accustomed signifies their emotional socialization.

Therefore, for children growing up within a family atmosphere prevalent with anger and aggression such as evident in inter-parental conflict, the children become socialized into anger. For such children, it will be easier to react to others in anger compared to children with minimal exposure to aggression or those exposed to an environment where parents adopt problem solving skills instead of anger. A study on socialization and children's development emotionally and socially indicated that parents behavior have some implication on children's emotional socialization (Baker, Fenning, & Crnic, 2011). For this reason, children that have supportive parents will have a greater opportunity to develop positive emotional and social function.

Children with poor social function show poor problem solving skills and have a challenge in appropriate interpretation of social cues. Such children tend to misinterpret their peers intentions, often thinking others intend them harm (DeBaryshe & Fryxell, 2013). The social learning process could explain the role of parental emotional response on children's emotional socialization (Mirabile, 2010). Through social learning, parents that show high levels of positive emotional response will likely promote a positive emotional climate for their children, in addition, helping them develop positive emotional expression (Mirabile, 2010). The parents that contain their emotional expressions will in turn teach their children that they should suppress their emotions rather than express them. Therefore, social learning suggests that parental emotional reactions will forge a path for adopted emotional behavior by their children. Based on the socialization argument, children exposed to high parental conflict could develop problems in addressing anger and will likely react with anger compared to children whose parents are less confrontational.

While research noted the potential for anger in relation to observation of marital conflict (Davies et al., 2006; DeBaryshe & Fryxell, 2013), literature on children's reaction to anger in adulthood is unavailable. This leaves a research gap relating to whether children will develop particular behaviors that they exhibit when presented with situations of anger. The behaviors are those that develop during their childhood as they observe the fights between their parents. The lack of literature presents an opportunity to explore the relationship between exposure to marital conflict and anger. The literature also does not provide a connection between anger and verbal marital conflict. This research, therefore, responds to a research gap on the impact of witnessing verbal marital conflict as a child and the behavior of anger responses as an adult. This research will provide empirical evidence on whether a connection exists between these variables.

## Significance of the Study

Bandura (1997) suggest through his social learning theory that even though the behavioral approach assist in not only understanding the anxiety and how to treat it, there is also the matter of the client's thought pattern, surroundings, and how it may affect the behavior of the client. Reinecke et al. (2003) mentions when diagnosing a client with violent behavior, the therapist should identify the client's schema and how it affects the cognitive behavior of the client. The schema will include the beliefs and view of the world through the eyes of the client. In order to determine any aggressive feelings from the client, the therapist should also develop skills that can be used to assess if the behavior is being modeled after the client's surroundings and environment to include family and social developments (Bustillos-Perez, 2011). Along with the training above, there are also four areas the therapist will use to build the skills necessary to target the emotionality of the client, which are: mindfulness skills, emotional regulations skills, distress tolerance skills, and interpersonal effectiveness skills (Linehan, 1987).

This study will benefit the participant, marriage, and family in that the research will focus on individual meaning and the importance of rendering the complexity of the situation. The information gathered will assist and benefit the participant in noticing if he/she was affected by the verbal marital conflict as a child and how the past may have affected their marital future. Hopefully, the participants will learn about themselves during the research and make the necessary changes to better their lives in their marriage, family, and all relationships. The research could help in the development of focused interventions for verbal marital conflict depending on the results.

The way a child learns how to handle conflict is learned in the household through observing the actions of the family (Feldman, Mashalha, & Derdikman-Eiron, 2010). If verbal marital conflict influences the development of anger responses in adults who witnessed the conflict as children measured by the Novaco Anger Scale (NAS; Novaco, 1994, 2003), then therapeutic designs and interventions should be created and utilized in order to protect the harm being placed on not only the external responses of the child/adult but also the internal responses.

An integration which can be used in the therapeutic design are behavioral counseling programs. There are cognitive behavioral programs in place used to treat abusive men. These programs (with modification) can also be effective in treating the behavioral anger responses in adults who witness marital conflict as children. Such techniques a therapist can use to treat an angry adult due to witnessing marital conflict as a child include: anger and stress management, communication training, and behavioral practices to include: self-monitoring, express calmly his/her verbal feelings to therapist and others involved, and discuss non-angry safety plans such as removing oneself from stressful situations (Babcock et al., 2004; Myers, 1995). The child/adult could possibly be harvesting or blocking ways to escape the emotions and reactions of witnessing marital conflict and this program could be useful in breaking those barriers. A cognitive behavioral program will not be physically used in the current study. However, cognitive behavioral programs will be touched upon in the dissertation as a therapy to assist in benefiting clients who seek therapy to deal with their anger issues due to witnessing marital conflict as a child.

This study may help therapists in understanding the impact of verbal marital conflict on adults' anger behavioral responses and explore that area when working with adults struggling with anger management. In addition, the results of this study may help therapists develop specific programs aimed at awareness raising activities for parents referred to child protection, etc. to help address such clinical concerns.

## Research Design

The study research design is a non-experimental/correlation using a survey to explore the relationship between witnessing verbal marital conflict as a child and adult behavioral responses of anger. The target group is adults with a targeted population of a minimum 100 participants for research through non-randomized sampling. The study does not involve any specification for the individuals involved in the responses. One consideration in the sampling process is that all the participants need to have witnessed verbal marital conflict as a child. The survey will seek responses concerning verbal conflict tactics and emotions on the anger response behavior in adults. The focus is on their developed behavior of anger according to the Novaco Anger Scale (NAS; 1994, 2003). The participants will sign a consent form agreeing to participate in the study. The survey delivery will be online, with a survey company assisting in reaching the participants. The online company SurveyGizmo provides an avenue for e-mailing and distribution of questionnaire to a specific audience selected by the researcher. An informed consent form will be made available before the survey can be accessed. Regarding the consent form, the participants are required to check a box to choose to participate or to not participate and the answer will show their willingness to participate in the study and their understanding of the consent form. The participants will receive instructions at the beginning of the survey. As the survey is self-administered, the participants will have the control over whether they want to complete the survey or not.

The study will use the Novaco Anger Scale (NAS; 1994, 2003), developed in 1994 and revised in 2003, which has a scale containing 60 items for self-reporting. The points included in the scale are cognitive, arousal, and behavioral. The scale describes anger through its connection to an individual. The level of measurement is ordinal. Another scale used in the study is the Children's Perception of Interparental Conflict scale developed in 1992 (CPIC; Grych et al., 1992). The Children's Perception of Interparental Conflict scale (CPIC; Grych et al., 1992) is a five-point, 49-item scale measuring the interparental conflict from the views of children. The categories included in the measurement are coping, self-blame, triangulation, stability, perceived threat, frequency, efficacy, intensity, resolution, and content. The study uses both scales in their entirety. The data analysis from the tools will be through Statistical Package for Social Studies (SPSS). The analysis of the Novaco Anger Scale (NAS; 1994, 2003) will be for only the behavioral subscale although the participants will have to complete the entire tool to avoid manipulation of participation.

## Research Questions and Hypotheses

The research question explored in this study is: What is the relationship between witnessing verbal marital conflict as a child and the behavior of anger responses as an adult?

*Ho:* There is no significant relationship between witnessing verbal marital conflict as a child and the behavior of anger responses as an adult.

*H:* There is a significant relationship between witnessing verbal marital conflict as a child and the behavior of anger responses as an adult.

## Assumptions and Limitations

An assumption of the study is that the researcher will be able to locate people willing to participate in the survey that experienced couple verbal conflict as children. Having an open inclusion criteria for the survey increases the likelihood of finding such participants.

Another assumption is that the participants will have recollections of their experiences in childhood and respond honestly to the survey. Recollection means that as an adult one will recall verbal confrontations between their parents and the effect this had on their well-being.

The study further contains the assumption that researcher will be able to make a connection between the participants witnessing verbal marital conflict as children with their responses to anger. Notably, a person could experience marital conflict in childhood and show no adverse interactions with anger in adulthood based on the Novaco Anger

Scale (NAS; 1994, 2003). However, if after taking the survey the participants do find a connection to their childhood witness and adult anger interactions, that they will seek counseling.

A limitation of the study is how to measure what entails a conflict. People may have different determinants of what they consider a conflict. For some, a mild confrontation between their parents could emerge as a conflict, while others consider instances of escalated shouting and probable violent gestures such as a person stomping out and banging the door. The study does use the Novaco Anger Scale (NAS; 1994, 2003), which provides indications of subscales of anger. The scale nonetheless shows elements entailed in anger response rather than the conflict. Considerations of how to defining a measurement for verbal conflict could be a potential research area. A definition will be provided on the survey defining verbal conflict.

Another limitation of the study is the risk involved with the study. No study is risk-free, however, there are minimal risk studies such as this one involving the recollection of childhood memories. There may be some participants who choose not to participant in the study or may choose not to finish the study because recalling the childhood memories of witnessing verbal marital conflict may be too much for the participant to face.

Using only the behavior subscale of the Novaco Anger Scale (NAS; 1994, 2003) may be seen as a limitation in the study; however, the participants will complete the scale in its entirety.

## Definitions of Terms

*Anger*. This refers to a reaction to irritation, which varies from intensity including mild irritation, frustration, and range (Anger Research Consortium, 2011). A person reacts in anger when they feel another is threatening them, their property, loved one, or a part of their identity. For example, a child intervening in the conflict of the parents could be because they feel the stronger parent is threatening the weaker one or the parent the child loves more. Anger may involve a physical reaction leading to a fight or running away. The reaction could be cognitive, referring to what a person thinks about the action leading to anger such as feelings of unfairness. Reference to anger in this study is on how adults as children that witnessed marital conflict respond to anger.

*Behavioral responses*. According to Novaco (2003), an important role used to define anger can be found through behavioral responses. To act in a confrontational manner towards a person or object supports the cognitive labeling of anger. Anger is most often viewed as a product of behavioral exchanges involving an escalation of aversive events, the behavioral manifestations of anger are critical dimensions for assessment and treatment. The NAS behavioral subscale is a combination of impulsive reaction, verbal aggression, physical confrontation, and indirect expression (Novaco, 2003).

*Child adjustment*. For this study, this refers to the ability of a child to fit within the circumstances of their life such as accepting the conflicts of the parents and moving beyond that conflict. It signifies the reaction of the child toward the conflict experience within the family (Towe-Goodman, Sifter, Coccia, Cox, and The Family Life Project Key

Investigators, 2011). A child that adjusts to the conflict finds a way to negate the negative implications of destructive conflicts.

*Child development*. This denotes holistic growth in the different areas of the progress of a child including emotionally, physically, and academically (Driscoll & Nagel, 2011). The focus of this study is the emotional development of a child faced with marital conflict. The study looks at how a child growing up with marital conflict is able to adjust and thus progress emotionally. This becomes evident in their ability to foster intimate relationships in future.

*Couples*. For this study, a couple will refer to two persons living together in agreement of having a marriage whether through a civil or religions certification. The people involved could be of different gender or same gender. The consideration is that the persons involved recognize themselves as a couple and with a family. The couple denotes two people connected by marriage or engagement and have a romantic relationship.

*Marital conflict*. This refers to interactions between a couple that involves differences in opinion characterized by verbal aggression, defensiveness, nonverbal hostility, personal insult, marital withdrawal, and physical aggression (Cummings & Davies, 2011). The conflict could be positive or negative depending on how the couple copes with the situation. When it involves aggression whether physical, verbal, or emotional it signifies the inability to resolve the situation amicable. Positive aspect involves communication and resolving the situation. The definition adopted in this study is the aggressive conflict involving married couples irrespective of the type of couple such as heterosexual and homosexual.

*Verbal conflict.* This is one area of marital conflict that involves a difference in opinions characterized by complaining, defensiveness, and confrontations as well as blame (Strong et al., 2011). Verbal conflict denotes spoken differences with each person in the relationship highlighting the problems they find in the other person. The definition adopted for this study is that verbal conflict involves finding fault noted through confrontations, without one accepting they could be at fault for the occurrences leading to the conflict.

## Expected Findings

The expectation of this study is to prove the alternative hypothesis is correct in that a significant relationship exists between witnessing verbal marital conflict as a child and the behavior of anger responses as an adult. The measurement of the Novaco Anger Scale (NAS; 1994, 2003) will indicate the relationship of anger behavior responses and the Children's Perception of Interparental Conflict Scale (CPIC; Grych et al., 1992) will indicate the relationship of conflict. Acknowledged in the study is that not all children will suffer due to verbal marital conflict, and depending on their social learning and emotional security their responses to anger may not be negative. However, the expectation is that some children may carry the emotional pain experienced as children who witnessed verbal marital conflict into their adulthood. This pain may then have a destructive part in their daily functioning and affect their lifestyle. Literature relating to the impact of marital conflict implies the destructive effect that undermines the quality of life the child has in later years such as in adulthood. Children unable to adapt to the conflict situation will continue to show maladaptive behavior in adulthood such as poor responses to instances of anger. This study will provide empirical evidence showing the impact of witnessing verbal marital conflict and the way the impact continues to affect a person even in adulthood. It responds to the established research gap showing whether people witnessing verbal marital conflict had definite anger responses based on the Novaco Anger Scale (NAS; 1994, 2003) that could have associations with their exposure to marital conflict as children.

## Organization of the Remainder of the Study

The study is described in this research proposal in four subsequent chapters. Following the introduction chapter will be the review of the literature, which will include the theoretical framework, gaps found in the existing literature, and an evaluation of the literature discussed in the study. The next chapter in the research study will focus on the methodology and research design used in the study. In addition, this section will also include a continuation of the purpose of the study, the target population, the procedures and instruments used to screen participants and collect data, the analysis of the data, ethical considerations, and the expected findings of the study. Next, the results chapter will give a description of the sampling procedure, summary of the results, and detailed information concerning the analysis and the results calculated by the data received from the participants. Tables containing statistical data will also be found in this chapter. The final chapter will discuss the results and conclusions of the study. Sections pertaining to limitations and future recommendations of the study can also be found in final chapter of the dissertation.

# CHAPTER 2. LITERATURE REVIEW

## Introduction to the Literature Review

The purpose of this research is to examine if there is a relationship between behavioral anger responses as adults after witnessing verbal marital conflicts in childhood. A considerable range of literature is available on the influence of inter-parental marital conflict on children. However, a gap still exists on the way the conflict continues to affect the children into adulthood. Through the literature review, it will be possible to substantiate this gap, identifying the elements left out in research that can be the focus of future studies while highlighting current knowledge on the subject. Included in the review is an overview of marital conflict, marital verbal conflict, influence on children, how the impact continues into adulthood, and establishing a theoretical framework for the research using emotional security theory (EST), and social learning theory (SLT), and then make an analysis on issues highlighted in the review and those the review leaves out.

The literature review follows the focus element proposed by Cooper (1988) in the "Organizing Knowledge Synthesis: A Taxonomy of Literature Reviews." Using the focus characteristic provides for the concentration on elements such as research outcomes, methods, theories arising in research, and application to practice and theory (Randolph, 2009). For this discussion, the focus is on empirical research findings on the way witnessing verbal marital conflict as a child affects behavioral anger responses in adulthood. This looks at whether researchers find a correlation between inter-parental conflicts with the children's anger responses in adulthood. When applicable the review further uses synthesis of literature or meta-analysis, depending on the focus of the synthesis and its relevance to the topic. The goal of the literature review is to find evidence in published literature or research on the way witnessing marital conflict influences children responses in adulthood, with focus on verbal conflict and anger responses as the main research variables. The literature review will provide a context for the current research as well as establish the existing research gap to show the significance of this research and need for new knowledge in the area of marital conflict and its influence on children and development.

## Theoretical Orientation for the Study

This section will explore the theories that will guide this study, emotional security theory (EST) and social learning theory (SLT). These theories further explain how marital conflict affects the socialization of children. SLT explores the aspect of children aping the actions they see the adults around them taking which could explain the socialization element of the study. The theory suggests that children who witness marital conflict can copy the behavior becoming aggressive and disruptive inside and outside the home (Bandura, 1969). EST reflects the emotional elements involved in children's response to the conflicts involving their parents (Davies & Cummings, 1994). The following section will identify the various elements involved in EST and SLT and where possible making connections to the discussion of marital conflict.

**Emotional Security Theory (EST)**

The theory arises from the recognition that couples have some level of conflict (Davies & Woitach, 2008). The problem arises when the disagreement grows into violence, disengagement, and unresolved conversations, therefore, creating an atmosphere of doubt for a person's safety and the concern may extend to the other members of the family including the children (Singh, 2010). EST explores the different attributes associated with the complex environment of conflicts among couples and finding solutions that would promote security for the family. The underlying argument in EST is that children feel safe or vulnerable depending on the conflicts occurring in the lives of their parents, and such conflicts trigger a social defense system in children (Davies & Woitach, 2008). Within the social defense system is an adoption of sets of behavior as coping mechanisms. The behaviors include fear, siding with one parent, becoming aggressive, distress, avoidance of conflicting situations, and inhibiting emotions where the children do not want to show their feelings. Another is trying to mediate over the situation by comforting the parents. The children could also become more sensitive to any threat that could come about during the conflict. When parents engage in conflicts, children develop response mechanisms that occur as the effect of the situation to their development. Depending on the constructive or destructive nature of the conflict, children will develop positive or negative coping behaviors.

EST derived from the work of Davies and Cummings (1994) to promote the understanding of how, when, and why conflicts between parents contribute to individual differences in the mental health trajectories of children. The developers posed the premise that conflict between parents poses a jeopardy to the modification of children by undermining their emotional safety with the parents, and compromising the attachment process of the child and parent through its connection with parenting commotions (Davies and Cummings, 1994). The research surrounding the initial work on EST showed two primary pathways explaining the risk posed by marital conflicts. The first was that the conflict increased the vulnerability of children in adjusting by progressively increasing their distress and reactivity to follow adult conflicts. The second interpretation was that conflict between parents acted as a link mediating the conflict with child psychological maladjustment.

Davies and Cummings (1994) promoted the idea that conflict between parents and accompanying disturbances in the family contributed to an emotionally charged experience for the children. Prior to this study, children were not primary participants in the conflict of their parents. The EST study considered a different approach where children would gain some form of primacy in the conflict. The theory connects attachment to security, but goes beyond attachment by stipulating that feeling secure with other family members was important. The attachment theory implied that when children feel stressed or treated badly, they maximize on the protection of their caregiver (Singh, 2010). The children express to the caregiver their distress, therefore, seeking comfort and ensuring they receive protection from the caregiver.

The differences seen in children in emotional security reflect the history of conflict among their parents. For example, families with continuous escalated conflicts will likely sensitize their children to have concern over their own security especially when the conflicts last for long and signify a possibility of other conflicts in the future (Singh, 2010). The conflicts damage the relationship of the children and their parents, and the solidity of the family. Children's concern about their security enables them to develop ways to cope with the threats arising from the parental conflict. For example, children that understand factors that trigger the conflict could try to avoid such triggers. Such an understanding contributes to children's involvement in the conflict

EST has key principles and pathways that explain the exposure of children to family discord and the differences in emotional security and psychological adjustment (Davies & Sturge-Apple, 2007). The principles include four groups, namely interparental discord defined by hostility, disengagement, and poor resolution (Davies & Sturge-Apple, 2007). The second is child emotional insecurity in the family characterized by interparental insecurity and parent-child security (Davies & Sturge-Apple, 2007). The third is child development trajectories of adjustment signifying the behavioral adjustment of children such as through adoption of externalizing and internalizing behaviors. The fourth is a group of family characteristics including parenting difficulties, family level processes, and child attributes. The fourth group of factors recognizes the variant of elements that contribute to conflict, possibility of coping, and outcomes in the children.

The goal of EST is to achieve emotional security in the lives of children. The reason comes from the belief that emotional security promotes mediation in the impact of parent and child attachment, promoting normal child development and development of psychopathology (Davies & Cummings, 1994). Additionally, when children feel secure in their attachment, their relationships extend beyond that of the immediate parent – child relationship to affect the adaptive functions in the grander social contexts and in other areas within the family.

EST extends to the feeling of security that couples could feel in their marriage. Based on attachment theory and extending to EST, when people marry they want to feel secure in their marriage where possible areas of security includes their thoughts, feelings, behaviors, and commitment. Marriage can also be a source of insecurity through conflicts and the way the couple handles them, which increases levels of insecurity and decreases satisfaction in the marriage. An insecure marriage is also a cause of stress for the couple especially when conflicts arise and the couple is unable to obtain amicable resolution to the conflict.

When a couple has a conflict, it extends even to those around them, reducing the emotional security experienced by others in the family such as the children. The children's emotional security relationship with the marital conflict is not due to the conflict or the reflected anger, but the connection it has on their feelings of security (Davies & Cummings, 1994). Emotional security provides a sense of what the conflict means for the family, and the quality of relationships in the family. Marital conflicts emotionally threatens children's feeling of security and any breakdown in the family worsens the situation. For example, if the conflict escalates to a level where the parents are no longer talking to each other, it signifies a breakdown in the family communication process and worsens the feelings of threat for the children.

Children can however learn how to manage the conflicts in their home through observation and participation. This leads to the social learning theory (SLT), which suggests how children learn in the family. Previously, the family arose as an agent of socialization, which contributes to the way children acquire behavior. The section on SLT shows the contribution of marital conflicts on children's lessons on coping.

**Social Learning Theory (SLT)**

This theory comes from the work of Bandura (1969) proposing that the process of socialization involves identificatory learning, with people acquiring behavior not through tuition, but by following observation of various socialization agents such as parents and peers. This explained that the acquisition of behavior had no reliable stimulus, but traced to cues presented by others surrounding the learner. Bandura (1969) explored the idea that social models acted as means to transmission and modification of behavior. This was denying the notion that behavior developed solely as an aspect of reward and punishment, and instead promoted the concept that emulating social behavior was a socially competent model of promoting learning.

To counteract the idea of reward and punishment, Bandura (1969) explained the absurdity of teaching language, familial customs of a culture, mores, vocational and avocational patterns, and its educational, social, and political practices through careful reinforcement without the reaction and assistance of models that exhibit accrued cultural repertoires. Such learning is short-circuited with other reinforcements presented through modeling having greater impact.

The disqualification of reinforcement through rewards and punishment does not mean that reinforcing behavior does not contribute to some form of learning. It rather signifies that the method has limitations because they signify laborious learning. For a person that finds it difficult to learn, it would mean continuous punishment for their errors. The limitations associated with the punishment and reward system undermines the effectiveness of reinforcement in learning behavior leading Bandura (1971) to suggest the concept of social learning where behavior acquisition is through modeling and socialization.

SLT denotes that behavior comes from learning the norms and values associated with the behavior such by participating in the activities or through observation (Siegel & Welsh, 2009). According to Siegel and Welsh (2009), the process of learning in SLT occurs within three subsets, namely differential association theory, differential reinforcement theory, and neutralization theory. The differential association theory refers to a subset developed by Edwin H. Sutherland in 1939 and finalized in 1947 that indicated behavior resulted from learning processes, and explaining that acquisition of behavior was a social learning process. A person learns by interaction with the people with the behavior they acquire. From them the learner gains values, attitudes, definitions, and other patterns of behavior. Differentiated association signifies learning, interaction, being an intimate part of the group, and attaining perceptions that influence motives and drives. Based on the period and frequency of the interaction, the level of influence will differ. This means that the longer a child interacts with a person the degree of influence will differ.

Neutralization theory involves a person acquiring and mastering the behaviors they want (Siegel & Welsh, 2009). This is possible by developing a set of values to explain behavior. A child will find excuses to explain away their bad behavior. The naturalization process can explain the reason why despite the socialization process some children adopt different values from those taught in the family.

SLT denotes that marital conflict affects children's development by providing an example behavior that children may adopt through modeling processes (Luster & Okagaki, 2011). The children observe their parents behavior seeing their negative strategies of conflict resolution and affective expressions. Such children are at risk of externalizing disorders and could become more aggressive toward their peers after seeing angry arguments between their parents. The anti-social behavior extends to their interactions with siblings, peers, and others close to them. Davies and Cummings (1994) explaining the impact of marital conflict on children noted that it affects children emotional responses. Notable in this study is the element of the learning behavior from parents. Children that observe their parents verbally abusing each other could become abusive to their peers and siblings unless they can decide purposively to adopt positive behavior. Bandura (1973) suggested that children who watched their parents' marital conflict learned the disorderly behavior and repeated it through externalization in their interactions with others. Some children through the emotional aspect of the interaction could blame themselves for the altercations between the parents and could develop guilt on the emotional level, while others would adopt the behavior through the socialization process. The frequency in which children observe their parents' confrontations promote internal non-adaptive conflict resolution that could later manifest through aggression, especially in children who have an emotional connection to the aggression. Consider for example a child that noted when one of their parents was verbally bullying the other, the one receiving became quite and grabbed something to hit the abusive partner. The child could perceive this as an accepted model of response. Therefore, marital conflicts could teach the child the behavior to adopt and the expected response.

The connection between EST and SLT is through the emotional effect of the parents' aggression toward each other, and the behavioral and psychological responses of the child. Some children will develop an aversive behavior to the pattern of abuse, while others will adopt the behavior depending on their emotional connectivity to the related actions (Davies & Cummings, 1994). The defense mechanisms and behavior adopted could become detrimental to the future of the children as they carry such connections to their adulthood. For some, they could become aggressive in future intimate relationships as an attribute of learned behavior. The patterns of behavior learned in childhood influence the future behavior adopted as the children mature into adults.

The connections made between children, marital conflicts, and forming maladaptive behavior focuses on marital conflict in general. This includes a range of conflicts including verbal, physical, and emotional (Cummings, 1998). The common ground is the aggressive nature of the conflict. This study considers the verbal marital conflict and its influences on child development. The theoretical foundations of the research, SLT and EST suggests that depending on the range of interaction and frequency, the adopted behavior will vary. This study does not consider the period of interaction but focuses on exposure to conflict, and its implications on child development. The concentration in research has further been directly on children. This study takes an alternate approach by looking at adults exposed to marital conflict as children. This creates a focal point beyond the influence of marital conflict within the period of occurrence to its implications beyond the years of childhood. The question to ask is whether people exposed to marital conflict as children experience challenges in adulthood especially in relation to behavioral anger responses. This widens the scope of focus for research in the effect of marital conflict on children (Cummings & Davies, 2002).

## Review of Research Literature and Methodological Literature
### Marital Conflict

In adulthood, people portray behaviors and seek help for behaviors that counselors or therapists trace back to the environment in which the individual grew-up in. For example, if an individual grew up in an abusive family then their behaviors as adults may also be abusive (Cummings & Davies, 2011; Nicholas & Rasmussen, 2006). The relationship of the behavior and the environment comes from classification of behaviors characteristic of people that grew up within certain family frameworks. Much focus has been on the adjustment of children to marital conflict or the effect conflicts in marriage have on children (Towe-Goodman, Sifter, Coccia, Cox, and The Family Life Project Key Investigators, 2011), although some researchers are looking at the long-term influence as the children approach adolescence and adulthood (Clarey, Hokoda, & Ulloa, 2010; Simon & Furman, 2010). To better understand the influence of marital conflict, an exploration of the phrase *marital conflict* is important.

A publication by Grych and Fincham (1990) called "Marital Conflict and Children's Adjustment: A Cognitive-Contextual Framework", provides a beginning point on understanding marital conflict, presenting a historical understanding of the phrase when research in the area was picking up. Grych and Fincham (1990) explain that all marriages have some degree of conflict, although not all qualify as stressful for children, but some conflict expose children to constructive problem-solving and coping strategies. Therefore, the impact of marital conflict relates to the type of conflict and its escalation level.

Agreeing with Grych and Fincham (1990), Cummings and Davies (2010) explain that marital conflict has both a negative and positive element, and can be an element of growth for the family when handled constructively. Marital conflicts become destructive when families and parties involved avoid them or withdraw. Strong, DeVault, and Cohen (2011) promote the same idea, identifying that happy marriages are not conflict free, the difference is in the way they handle conflict by using positive strategies, while unhappy marriages have negative ways of handling conflict. Strong et al. (2011) introduce the concepts of destructive and constructive conflicts, denoting that marital conflict becomes destructive when the parties are unable to resolve it or it continues to heightened proportions.

Marital conflict refers to a situation characterized by significant levels of verbal conflict, distrust, poor communication, anger, and cooperation such as in parenting, and an ongoing harmful attitude toward one's partner (McIntosh, 2010). The partners may show covert or overt hostility toward each other or project rude accusations pertaining to the other partner such as how the other partner parents the child. Conflicting parents further show threatening behaviors toward each other and the threats could escalate into violence when unresolved. In high conflict situations, verbal conflicts can grow into physical conflicts that pose a risk to the parties involved and their children.

Moving from the high conflict scenario of McIntosh (2010), Cummings and Davies (2011) pursue the definition of marital conflict in both major and minor interactions. They define marital conflict as any major or minor inter-parental interaction involving differences of opinion and can be positive or negative. Adapting this definition for Cummings and Davies (2011) was significant in addressing a wider range of marital behaviors including verbal aggression, defensiveness, nonverbal hostility, marital withdrawal, personal insult, and physical aggression on the negative side of the marital conflict spectrum. On the positive side, the authors could consider support, affection, and problem solving as part of conflict. This brought together considerations of conflict and conflict management or response, as both elements have implications on the way the conflict will affect the children in the relationship.

Expounding on marital conflict, Edleson and Nissley (2011) present the idea of domestic violence and exposure naming domestic violence exposure for children to include physical violence, verbal and emotional. The authors adopt a description to domestic violence exposure useful in this research. It refers to multiple experiences children experience when living at home where an adult uses violent conduct in a coercive repetition against an intimate partner according to Edleson and Nissley (2011). The definition extends to heterosexual and homosexual intimate partners, as both groups form families in the current society.

Surfacing in this section is that marital conflict has two extremes, destructive and constructive, which are part of the definitional paradigm. Destructive marital conflict refers to conflict characterized by behaviors such as avoidance, inflexibility, escalating spirals including manipulation, threats and coercion, retaliation, competition, and insulting verbal and nonverbal communication (Strong et al., 2011). Persons involved in a destructive conflict further exhibit behaviors such as criticizing, defensiveness, complaining, confrontation, and contempt of the other person. In contrast, a constructive conflict will involve adoption of communication traits such as clarification, and validating. Cummings and Davies (2010) points out the traits of support, affection, and problem solving as aspects of positive conflict.

Ultimately, destructive conflict causes distress in families and hampers interactions among parents and between parents and their children (Cummings & Davies, 2010). Conflict affects every member of the family especially when those involved cannot find an amicable resolution. In some instances, parents could be having a conflict but others in the family are unaware of it (Nicholas & Rasmussen, 2006). The notable element is that the impact of marital conflict extends to a level where other members of the family can become part of that conflict whether emotionally or physically. The implications of marital conflict on children in the short-term and long-term will essentially reflect the level of exposure the child had to his or her parents' conflicts. Higher levels of exposure to destructive conflict could have negative implications compared to lower exposure or exposure mainly to positive elements of inter-parental conflicts.

**Verbal Conflict.** Verbal conflict is a subset of marital conflict evident in the way, a couple undergoing a conflict chooses to articulate their differences in opinion. Definition of verbal conflict reflects the elements of constructive versus destructive marital conflict. Strong et al. (2011) identifies three elements that define verbal conflicts in distressed married couples, namely confrontation, defensiveness, and complaining. In confrontation, both partners confront each other, with each blaming the other for the problem or issue under discussion (Strong et al., 2011). The partners use phrases such as "You are the one who is wrong!" "It's not my fault, but yours!" Confrontation involves finding fault with the other, without accepting any part of the responsibility (Strong et al., 2011). In destructive conflict, none of the partners accepts blame or takes responsibility, but instead will find justification for their action moving to the second element, defensiveness (Strong et al., 2011).

The partner on the receiving end of the confrontation becomes defensive, suggesting they took a certain action in response to the action of their partner. For example, a person could say, "You did it first! I was only responding!" or "I only did what I was supposed to do, after what you did!" In both cases, the partner is using the action of the other partner to justify their recourse. In connection to defensiveness is complaining, where one partner or both complain about the others lack of a positive response (Strong et al., 2011). For example, one may say, "This is the best I can do without any help!" suggesting the other is not helpful. Verbal conflict becomes destructive when partners use mainly negative comments or statements in reference to the other partner such as the examples provided (Strong et al, 2011).

Positive verbal conflict involves use of statements through paraphrasing, clarification, validation, and summarizing with a positive impact on the conversations (Strong et al., 2011). For example, a person could clarify the point made by the other prior to making a negative comment or interpretation, such as by asking, "could you please explain what you mean so that I understand you." Using such a phrase will create an avenue for better dialogue, or even paraphrasing by putting what the other said as a way of creating deeper understanding. For example, one partner could say, "what you are saying is that I am not a good listener." This ensures both parties are aware of the nuances of the discussion without taking offense. Clarey et al. (2010) confirm that constructive conflict involves trying to make the situation better by discussing the problem with the person who is the object of the anger. This is in contrast to behaving aggressively toward the person or misdirecting the anger to someone outside the immediate conflict as is characteristic of destructive conflict.

For the purpose of this research, the focus is on destructive conflict and destructive comments that partners make in intimate relationships or in a marriage. The assessment is on how such statements could have a long-term effect on their children. The assumption is that the children are present in such confrontations and are aware of the ongoing battle between their parents. Another assumption is that the conflict is not a one-time occurrence in the family but a recurrent problem. The assumption is that for a destructive conflict to have a lasting impact on the members of the family, it is frequent and characterized by hostile and negative interaction such as what is evident in heated arguments, name calling, insulting, failing to listen, and display of unemotional attachment. Exposure for children, therefore, is on the frequent and negative attributes of their parents' relationship.

**Marriage, Family, and Child Socialization.** An area significant to this discussion is identifying that the marital conflict occurs within a family setting, where a couple has a child or children and the child feels the occurring altercation. The couple could be heterosexual, homosexual or any other form of a couple. The significant element is that the interaction of the couple has a bearing on the children and the family. The consideration is that marital conflict suggests a couple is living together in some form of marriage or a family.

The family begins the socialization process through which children learn and develop to be the person they become in adulthood (Akers, Krohn, Lanza Kaduce, & Radosevich, 1979; Bandura, 1973; Driscoll & Nagel, 2011). For example, when you meet a person and later his or her family, it becomes possible to understand the person's behavior. For children brought up in an aggressive home and they develop aggressive tendencies, meeting their family explains the beginning point of such tendencies. However, this does not mean it will be true for every person as others develop behavior central to their upbringing. This does not mean the family did not act as a socialization agent; it just signifies an opposite effect where the person chooses to adopt other behaviors and values differing from those of their family.

The family as a socialization agent forms the first contact in which a child will learn values, behaviors, and begin their psychosocial development (Driscoll & Nagel, 2011). The effect of the family unit is stronger in the initial years of child development but begins to diminish as the child attends preschool, and other programs. Plus, school begins to influence child's development. Nonetheless, the family is the origin of developing trust, independence, initiative, competence, self-esteem, decision-making capabilities, and developing the mechanisms enabling building and nurturing of a relationship with others.

In the family, children acquire moral ethics and social principles through socialization. The procedure involves a multifaceted interchange between evolutionary biases and hereditary and socio-cultural factors. The role of the parents is diverse and parents foster it through a parent and child relationship. The parents' role includes protecting their children, mutual exchange, controlled management, steered learning, and helping them participate in different activities (Grusec, 2011). Parents help their children mainly by being supportive and understanding their experiences. By having some degree of controlled management over their own actions parents help build their character.

Based on the socialization effect of the family, when the family presents an aggressive front to the child, the child will tend to identify with aggression (Driscoll & Nagel, 2011). The socialization process could be unintended where the parents did not perceive their conflict as having an effect on the child's socialization. The intentional nature of socialization may not have a critical bearing on the behavior of the child due to the child's capacity to copy from their family (Akers et al., 1979; Bandura, 1973; Driscoll & Nagel, 2011). For example, while during an argument the couple call each other names, such as one telling the other they were worthless and did not know how to do anything. Even though the statement should not be meaningful to the children, they pick up the intonation, beginning to think of the other parent as worthless. If the abused parent was the mother, the children could take the lesson further to mean that the female gender is worthless. The parents could be telling the children to value every person irrespective of their difference, but their interactions with each other contradict the positive message.

An example of marital conflict socialization aspect, when children witness intense conflict between the parents they could adopt aggressive behavior, while children that witness constructive instances even in conflict learn how to handle conflict. For example, when parents talk about their differences and resolve them appropriately, children understand that relationships have conflicts but it is possible to resolve them amicably. They obtain constructive problem-solving skills that they can use in solving their conflicts in the future (Faircloth, 2012). Viewing constructive conflict helps strengthen the children's logic of safety in the family as a foundation of solidity, receptiveness, and love (Faircloth, 2012). Marital conflict can be a source of promoting both positive and negative learning environments for children depending on the way the parents use the conflicts. To facilitate positive socialization, marital conflict should be constructive to predict positive outcomes or counter the negative that could lead to antisocial behaviors and psychological challenges in children (Faircloth, 2012). Constructive socialization promotes pro-social behavior, lowers the incidences of psychological problems and increases the self-esteem of children (Faircloth, 2012). It also promotes emotional security as children experience warmth from the parents.

**Implications of Marital Conflict on Children Adjustment.** A myriad of research exists indicating the negative impact of marital conflict on children adjustment for infants (Dejonghe, Bogat, Levendosky, von Eye, & Davidson, 2005), pre-school age children (Towe-Goodman et al., 2011), adolescents (Simon & Furman, 2010; Clarey et al., 2010; Simon & Furman, 2010), and into adulthood (Cannon, Bonomi, Anderson, Rivara, & Thompson, 2010). The studies, which are a blend of quantitative and qualitative designs, provide evidence that marital conflict acts as a determining factor for future behavior among these anger and perpetration of anger, as well as being a recipient of violence in interpersonal relationships.

The reason marital conflict affects children, is that they are active participants of the conflict even though they may not interact directly with the couple during the aggression (Buehler, 2014). Their participation is through observation, hearing, and sensing the exchanges between the couple or feeling the tension. The children react to the conflict and make interpretations sometimes taking the blame. Therefore, although adults may not perceive the children as part of their confrontations, their presence within the relationship make them active participants. The following discussion recognizes the different areas where marital conflict in its various forms affects the well-being of children and their development.

**Intergenerational Transmission of Conflict.** Kerley, Xu, Sirisunyaluck, and Alley (2010) in their study on exposing family violence and victimization or perpetration of violence in adulthood, began by noting that having a history of family violence acts as a predisposing factor to subsequent offending and victimization in adult life. Adults that grew up under direct exposure to conflict in the family; such as they experienced violence or witnessed violence against a member of the family, will likely show violent tendencies later in adulthood. An intergenerational transmission research using a sample containing 816 married women from Thailand provide evidence on how childhood exposure to violence initiates a future of partner perpetration and victimization according to Kerley et al. (2010). The women showed that exposure to household violence in childhood had an indirect impact on their mental, emotional, and bodily intimate partner perpetration, but a direct association of parental partner violence with psychological and physical victimization in adulthood (Kerley, et al., 2010).

In another study on women using a randomized sample of 3,568 women, the researchers assessed the impact of childhood exposure to intimate partner violence (IPV) and child abuse on women's health, adult IPV, and the use of healthcare services (Cannon et al., 2010). The study findings indicated that compared to women that had not had exposure to IPV, those with exposure to IPV had greater use of healthcare services for mental health, had worse health outcomes, and a higher prevalence of depression especially for those that experienced both intimate partner violence and abuse. Women experiencing only intimate partner violence had adverse long-term and incremental effects on health and relationships. Cannon et al. (2010), and Kerley et al. (2010) studies show the possible continuation of conflicts in interpersonal relationships. The suggestion is an intergenerational transmission of conflict, where those persons that experienced inter-parental conflict as children have a heightened likelihood of experiencing conflict in their intimate relationships as adults. The experience as emerging from Kerley et al. (2010) can be as victims or perpetrators.

Clarey et al. (2010) give evidence of violence perpetration for those exposed to marital conflict in childhood. Using a sample of 204 high school students, the study investigated the relationships of teen dating violence to exposure to inter-parental violence, anger, and acceptance of violence. Using regression analysis, the survey conducted among teenagers from Monterrey, Mexico revealed that teens who grew up in families that accepted violence beliefs and anger, and inter-parental conflict; their interpersonal relationships would have dating violence with the exposed teen as the perpetrator. The dilemma was having problems with anger control which was an aspect learned from the parents; hence, the teen would be imitating the parents' behavior and acceptance of violence within the family.

The experiences and perceptions attributed to the inter-parental conflicts would reflect in the way a person interacted with others in their romantic relationships. In a study of 183 senior high school students responding to a questionnaire and 88 observations, it was evident that the adolescents' perception and appraisal of inter-parental conflict, which related the amount of conflict and conflict styles, moderated the adolescents' romantic relationship (Simon & Furman, 2010). The suggestion resulting from the study is that exposure to inter-parental conflict and the meanings the children ascribe to the conflict will contribute to their future relationship experiences.

In her study, Turcotte-Seabury (2010) examines the mediating effect between exposure to inter-parental conflict and perpetration of violence with limited anger management. The study that comprised 14,252 students and multinomial logistic regression analysis, showed that participants who experienced inter-parental violence reported higher levels of perpetrating violence and they had more limited anger management abilities compared to those unexposed to inter-parental conflict. Having limited anger management abilities also had a positive association with violence perpetration. The study reflects the findings of Kerley et al. (2010), Clarey et al. (2010), and Simon and Furman (2010) that exposure to inter-parental conflicts increased the likelihood of a person engaging in interpersonal conflicts in the future with those exposed as violent perpetrators. However, the study adds the dimension of anger to engagement in conflict, suggesting that the inability to deal with anger increased possible perpetration of violence. Clarey et al. (2010) had a similar view that anger control issues linked to future violence. As indicated by Turcotte-Seabury (2010) and Clarey et al. (2010), learned behavior in anger management is an element in future association with intimate relationship violence. Therefore, research suggests there is an intergenerational transfer of conflict conduct from parent to child, where exposure to conflict predisposes the child to adopting a conflict strategy in future relationships as adolescents and adults.

**Effect of Marital Conflict on Children in Various Age Groups.** When couples have a conflict, it affects children of all ages (Faircloth, 2012), beginning with children as young as six months old and up to adolescence (The Tavistock Center for Couple Relationships (TCCR), 2014). For example, babies show psychological symptoms of distress when exposed to a hostile interaction between their parents (TCCR, 2014). The distress is evident through increased heart rate. This finding is in contrast to experienced hostility between non-parental adults. For infants and children up to five years of age, the children show their distress through crying, withdrawing from their parents, or acting out.

Sometimes they could attempt to intervene in the conflict. Children from six years up to 17 years of age also exhibit emotional and behavioral distress when faced with parents acrimonious exchanges. These findings indicate that children of varying age groups suffer anxiety and distress over their parents' acrimony. Other manifestations of children responses are: becoming aggressive to their peers and others, showing hostility even to people trying to intervene in their situation, and adopting anti-social behavior. Some children begin to perform poorly in school and could become juvenile delinquents.

In a study conducted by the University of Notre Dame and the University of Rochester, the researcher showed that kindergarten aged children exposed to marital discord develop long-term emotional problems that could manifest in adolescence (Nauert, 2012). The study, conducted over seven years, involved 235 mothers, fathers, and children from a middle-class background (Nauert, 2012). Results of the study showed that over the study period, the children developed emotional security in the early school years and continued emotional challenges in adolescence (Nauert, 2012). Implications from the study were that children exposed to parental discord had a higher probability of developing emotional insecurity in later childhood, and during adolescence they would develop problems in adjustment with possible emotional challenges being depression and anxiety (Nauert, 2012). The reason is that conflict denied the children emotional security in the family. A secure family promotes safety, protection, and security affecting the emotional and social dimensions of the children.

Historical indications on conflicts between parents was that parental acrimony was a threat to children when overt and mostly violent, but it is becoming evident that even when the conflict is verbal and non-violent it could lead to negative effects on the development of children (Rhoades, 2008). Research suggested that conflicts did not have to be violent, but it instead range from silent to violent, and ranging on the severity, it produced a certain degree of a negative effect on children (Cummings & Davis, 2010). An example of how silent acrimony affects children is when parents withdraw emotionally from one another. The lack of warmth and affection affects children's emotional development, and could affect their relationships in the future.

Evidence is lacking on whether marital conflict affects babies younger than six months, as the available research shows six months to 17 years of age (Rhoades, 2008). Based on such age findings, one can conclude that conflict between couples can lead to psychological and behavioral challenges to children across a large spectrum. When considering the implications on children by age, an evolving aspect is that their coping will depend highly on their age. For example, the impact on younger children will depend on the capacity of the child to process the activity; whereas, that of the older child will depend on their secondary processing (Rhoades, 2009). The reason is that as children grow their responses stop depending on egocentric and catastrophic attributes and become sophisticated. This could explain why depression cases may arise with increase in age. Younger children have a greater likelihood of accepting blame for the events and feeling the threat attributed to the conflict. For older children, their dysfunction will relate to their cognitive attributes.

However, Rhoades (2009) notes that the role played by age remains unclear in children's responses to conflict between couples. This presents a possible area of future research where researchers would consider the relationship between age and the effect of marital conflicts. The studies could look at whether the age of the child contributed to the possible impact of the conflict on their behavior and emotional well-being. The indications presented in this section seem to indicate that younger children will suffer psychologically and have a greater likelihood to blame themselves while older children have less concern but could develop behavioral problems. The older children develop coping mechanisms that enable them to avoid the conflict when possible; although they will continue to feel its impact on their lives despite avoidance.

Johnson (2009) noted that children's behavior relating to internalization or externalization varied on the circumstances and age of the child. For example, among four to nine year old children, couple conflict led to internalizing behaviors among children. However, the author noted that the relationship between age, behavior, and couple conflict remains unclear. The reason is double-sided results showing significant correlation and others showing age is not a significant factor. Therefore, the issue of age remains unclear. The current study is not specific to any age group but looks at children in general without dividing them into groups. Considerations of age would be beyond the scope of this study at this time.

**Anger Management and Control.** Through a developmental perspective on anger, DeBaryshe and Fryxell (2013) noted that emotional socialization begins at childhood, and children exposure to anger comes from seeing their parents' anger or that of people around them. From this exposure, children develop models of anger and conflict resolution models based on the lessons acquired. Through emotional socialization, children form reactive models even for anger and emotional management, which affects their interactions with their peers and determine their aggressive versus pro-social peer interactions (DeBaryshe & Fryxell, 2013). The ability to form close relationships depend on their management skills for dealing with anger and emotions developed following exposure to interparental anger. When children venture into the social world, the lessons learned at home accompany them including experiences of anger and aggression. The interaction they formed during family socialization forms the basis of their interaction patterns with others. In lieu of socialization, children socialized into anger will have a greater propensity of reacting with others with anger compared to children socialized into an environment where others adopt problem-solving skills rather than anger. Children oriented into anger could also become targets for unprovoked aggression.

Children that have a tendency for anger have poor social problem solving skills and find it challenging to attend to social cues, misinterpret intentions among their peers, and often think others intend harm (DeBaryshe & Fryxell, 2013). Another aspect increasing the potential challenges of anger is that the children exposed to verbal conflict have information processing deficits therefore failing to interpret positive and negative emotions among their peers (Faircloth, 2012). The indications is that they face challenges in interpretation of pro-social intentions and gauge their reaction to pro-social events. When others show them positive behavior, they feel surprise as this is not expected. A consideration to make is that children subjected to extreme degrees of parental conflict will have greater challenge with anger and management of anger compared to those with lower levels of aggression in their live (Bauer et al., 2006; Davies & Cummings, 1994). Further, persons exposed to high confrontations at home will be less likely to show upset when facing the same issues outside the home. The reason is familiarity with such situations at the family level.

***Behavioral Anger Response.*** The research on the influence of verbal marital conflict and interparental conflict on behavioral anger response in children and adults is highly lacking. An electronic database search and Google search for behavioral anger responses, and behavioral anger response and interparental conflict failed to yield findings relevant to the discussion even when adding the elements of children and adults to the search parameters. A search on interparental conflict and anger response in the Academic Full Search database yielded one useful research, but it was published more than a decade previously. The article highlighted that interparental verbal conflict caused a variant of reaction among children. These reactions included sadness, anger, and guilt contingent on the age of the child (Adamson & Thompson, 1998). For children exposed to violent interparental conflict, they tended to have greater anger response compared to others therefore showing children's sensitivity to conflict within the home.

Kassinove (2014) provides direction on recognition of anger. Kassinove (2014) defines anger as a state associated with hostility and maladaptive behavior developed in response to the unwanted actions of others that a person perceives as demeaning, sees as lacking respective, or feels is threatening. Based on the hostility and maladaptive behavior, a person may seek revenge. Anger response is an interpretation of the behavior of others which comes from seeing malevolence in others leading to distorted interpretations (Lochman, Barry, Powell, & Young, 2010). The implication is that a person will tend to react to the perceived malevolence in anger and sometimes in hostility. This shows that behavioral anger response is a consequence of interpretation, although, the literature does not provide adequate connection to parental or verbal marital conflict. In addition, recent research is unavailable showing children and adult behavioral anger response to various stimulation such as verbal marital conflict.

**Effect on Future Romantic Relationships.** Children coming from backgrounds with marital conflict could have problematic future relationships. Yu, Pettit, Lansford, Dodge, and Bates (2010) conducted a study on the main effect and interactive models of the relations between marital conflict among other issues and the effect on the child's relationship with others including parent and adult child relationship. The results showed that marital conflict was a cause of poor quality of parent – adult child relationship. The child creates a negative attribution to one parent such as the mother, with the most affected people being women. The findings of the study signify that conflict creates problematic relationships for the child even as they approach adulthood. The problematic relationship is not only on the intimate aspect but also on their relationship with the parents. As noted previously, children may undermine the parent on the receiving end of the abuse. For example, if the father usually abuses the mother, then the child could undermine the place of the mother in their lives. The mother becomes less important. Alternatively, if the child feels the father or abusive parent is in the wrong, then the child could undermine the role of the parent. The implication of the study is that the marital conflict affects the quality of relationships that the child will have in the future even as they attain adulthood.

Yu (2007) in another study found a relationship between growing up with parents with marital conflict. Yu (2007) found a relationship between witnessing marital conflict and multiple problems. The problems included the potential for treating a future partner with contempt, having conflicts in the relationship, and being unable to sustain relationships. The explanation is that the children develop insecurity in their romantic relationships undermining the quality of the relationship. Although the study combined the issue of divorce and marital conflict, it provided evidence on the relationship on conflict and relationship quality in the future. The poor relationship quality and possible dissolution of intimate relationships occurs when the children have a more positive attitude toward the behavior they saw among their children (Cui, Fincham, & Durtschi, 2010). For example, a child who saw poor commitment in the marriage of their parents will have a poor view of commitment and may withdraw from the relationship if it demands much from them. The development of a romantic relationship and its possible dissolution depends on the behavioral adjustment of the child. For example, children who are able to find coping mechanisms due to the conflict between their parents, may be able to support a healthy relationship. Behavioral adjustments show that the child has been able to accept the relationship between their parents and move beyond the conflict. Cui et al. (2010) indicated that the family can act as a point of explaining the quality of relationships that people have and their dissolution. The commitment of children to their future relationships will reflect their socialization on commitment to romantic relationships. For example, a study conducted by Miga, Gdula, and Allen (2011) indicated that inter-parental relationships predicted the satisfaction of their children in their romantic relationships up to seven years following exposure. The reason is that the parental actions influence the behavior of their children and approaches borrowed by the children. Adaptability and achievement of a constructive romantic relationship could indicate the parents having impacted on the child a possible avenue to resolve conflict.

***Behavioral Problems.*** A research area in the effect of marital conflict on children is on children's behavioral outcomes. Rhoades (2009) found that children exposed to conflict between their parents developed behavioral problems associated with the conflict. The categories of behavior for children witnessing marital conflict are involvement and avoidance behaviors. Involvement behavior refers to activities that will try to stop the conflict such as talking to the parents during the conflict or interrupting them physically when they are arguing (Fosco & Grych, 2008). Avoidance behaviors involve children trying to avoid their parents actively during the conflict when they are aware that the parents are arguing (Fosco & Grych, 2008). These are immediate reactions of children during the conflict of the couples in their lives. Moreover, it marks the beginning point of their reactions to conflicts. Avoidance acts as an indicator of internalization of behavioral problems later (Fosco & Grych, 2008). The avoidance tactics adopted by the child will however signify whether the marital conflict will lead to a negative or positive affect (Fosco & Grych, 2008). For example, for children who avoid the conflict by engaging in some positive activity or adopting coping mechanism, they are likely to avoid the negative effects compared to those who remain connected to the conflict. The potential implications of the conflict on the child relates to the responses of the child.

Through a meta-analysis, Rhoades (2009) found that the effect of cognitions and internalization behavior problems were considerably grander to those of behavioral and physiological responses. Comparisons for behavior internalization or externalization indicated that many behavioral problems showed internalization. Further exploration of internalization and externalization indicated that marital conflict affects children's psychological functioning especially through exposure of recurrent occurrences of destructive conflict (Faircloth, 2012). Depending on the degree of destructiveness it can cause internalizing problems such as unhappiness and low self-confidence; as well as externalizing behavioral problems such as criminal behavior, anger, decline in academic performance, social and interpersonal modification, and broad mental health encounters (Faircloth, 2012). Children exposed to constant marital conflicts suffer health related risks including emotional health.

One need not assume that because of constant exposure to conflict children become used to it. Rather than gaining tolerance, the children become sensitized to the conflict exposing them to its impact (Faircloth, 2012). They then have a lower threshold for exposure to agony and anger leading them to become extremely provoked during a disagreement. This means that even a mild disagreement causes distress. The children show emotional distress including fear, anger, and sadness leading from the conflict. If the parents were able to address their conflicts constructively it could be more beneficial to the child, showing them how to address future conflicts. The family acts a significant acceptance for violence in intimate relationships.

## Summary of the Literature Review

Based on the findings in the literature review, marital conflict affects the development of children. It seems marital conflict affects the emotional development of children and they adopt internalization and externalization behaviors in reaction to the conflict. Marital conflict signifies the inability of parents to resolve their differences and the children are active participants of the conflict. Though the children may not be in the conflict, they participate by observation and sometimes trying to intervene in the altercation. Aligning to the emotional security theory (EST), witnessing marital conflict exposes children to a feeling of insecurity where they feel their parents are not able to protect them from what is occurring in the family. The exposure goes further by leading to learned behavior as suggested by social learning theory (SLT). The child picks up behaviors from their parents feeling that altercations between a couple is acceptable.

The literature review effectively shows the elements surrounding marital conflict and its impact on children and their development. However, the literature review shows a gap in available research regarding verbal conflict and anger responses. The available literature displays anger response as an attribute of stimuli from interpretation of perceived malevolence. Recent literature in the area of anger response published in the last five years is lacking, and the available literature does not provide adequate connection between behavioral anger response and exposure to verbal marital conflict. Lacking in the literature is the effect of verbal conflict on children and adults, and on anger response. Some reference to verbal conflict appears in the literature but direct studies are lacking. This presents an opportunity for future studies where researchers can explore the impact of direct exposure to specific types of marital conflict such as verbal conflict. The main focus in literature has been about physical violence. Another noticed gap in literature is on the impact of marital conflict on adults exposed to conflict as children. The focus in literature is on children, however, leaving a gap for researchers to examine the impact on adults that faced conflict between their parents. Another gap is on anger response on how persons exposed to marital conflict respond. This study explores the relationship between witnessing verbal marital conflict as a child and behavioral anger responses in adulthood.

# CHAPTER 3. METHODOLOGY

The study design was a non-experimental, correlational design using two survey tools for the data collection. This section explains the data collection design identifying the various benefits and considerations to make under the techniques and procedures employed. This chapter highlights the research procedure and sampling and restates aspects such as the purpose of the study, research questions and the hypothesis.

## Purpose of the Study

The purpose of the study was to explore the relationship between witnessing verbal marital conflict as a child and the behavior of anger responses as an adult. The researcher identified whether adults exposed to verbal marital conflict as children had behavioral responses of anger as adults based on the Novaco Anger Scale (NAS; 1994, 2003).

## Research Design

The study research design was a non-experimental/correlational design using two surveys. As a non-experimental survey, the researcher had the opportunity to interview participants through a questionnaire based on experiences. In this study the researcher explored the relationship between witnessing verbal marital conflict as a child and adult behavioral responses of anger. Non-experimental/correlation designs are ideal for studies that do not require manipulation of an independent variable (Berg & Latin, 2008). In the present study, the focus was on experiences of the participants rather than observing their response to established stimuli making the non-experimental design adequate. In addition, the researcher did not assume a cause effect relationship of experiencing verbal marital conflict as a cause for behavioral anger response. The objective of the research was to explore if witnessing verbal marital conflict during childhood could possibly play a role in anger responses as an adult in relationships and daily life experiences. The research would in no way introduce new experiences to the participants but test solely their experience as children and exposure to verbal marital conflict. The purpose of the study does not require an experiment to attain data which can effectively be collected based on the responses to the established questions of the surveys being used.

The target for this study was to identify 66 participants who could respond to two surveys. The participants had to be adults who experienced verbal marital conflict as children. The sample of 66 was large enough to provide a representative sample for the study. The sample size of 66 provided a minimal margin of error (Davis & Gallardo, 2010). The lower the sample size, the higher the margin of error. The more similar the population, the smaller the margin of error. Therefore, researchers are able to use a relatively small sample when the target population is similar (Quarles, 2001). The sampling was non-random to ensure the researcher was able to obtain a sample which fit within the characteristics sought. Using a non-random sampling is efficient for a researcher wanting a specific group or to attain a specific perspective that may not be well outlined using random sampling (Leedy & Ormrod, 2010).

The research questionnaire was a combination of the Novaco Anger Scale (NAS; 1994, 2003) and Children's Perception of Interparental Conflict (CPIC; Grych et al., 1992). The NAS (1994, 2003) is a 60-item self-reporting survey that tests cognitive, arousal, and behavioral responses. Although the participants are required to answer the entire survey to avoid manipulation of participation, only the behavioral subscale was used in the data analysis. The CPIC (Grych et al., 1992) is a 49-item scale that tests how children view interparental conflict in the following categories: coping, self-blame, triangulation, stability, perceived threat, frequency, efficacy, intensity, resolution, and content (Grych et al., 1992). Accompanying the questionnaire was a consent form that all participants had to agree to before proceeding with the study. The consent was an indication of willing participation in the study. An online company delivered the questionnaire and consent form by sending the participants an e-mail with the link to the research study. The survey company, SurveyGizmo has distribution options where it sends potential participants an e-mail based on the specifications provided by the researcher. Participants followed the research study link provided in their e-mail to participate. Once the required number of participants were documented, the data analysis from the two surveys was calculated through the Statistical Package for Social Studies (SPSS) to correlate if there was a relationship between the two variables.

## Target Population and Participant Selection

According to Stratus and Gelles (1990) 12% of American households experience some form of marital violence, and every year nearly 10 million children witness that violence. However, current research performed by Smith Slep and O'Leary (2005) shows a pattern of aggression can be found among married people who have at least one young child in the home. Based on the information provided in the partners' reports of this study, 49% of the couples reported physical aggression while 24% reported dangerous physical aggression (El-Sheikh, Cummings, Kouros, Elmore-Staton, & Buckhalt, 2008). In conjunction with this current research, El-Sheikh et al. (2008) notes the statistics seem to be higher in couple aggression than earlier reports and underestimated numbers when looking at the percentage of children open to the elements of marital violence. A more recent study done by McDonald et al. (2006) shows 30% of children (15.5 million) live in an environment where marital violence has taken place, and 13.3% of children live in an environment where severe violence has taken place in the past 12 months. Police reports have found that 44% of domestic violence occurred while children were present and 58% of the children present in these circumstances were under six years old. The statistics for children directly in the path of marital violence acts totaled 87% (Cummings, El-Sheikh, Kouros, & Buckhalt, 2009).

Little research has been produced linking race/ethnicity and child functioning (or outcomes) in children raised in high conflict homes, and studies searching for ethnic differences in aggressive marriages are turning up with inconsistent results (Cummings et al., 2009). Gelles (1993) reports an increase of marital violence can be found in African American families in comparison to European American families. However, Vogel and Marshall (2001) find no difference between African American families and European American families when socioeconomic status (SES) is placed in the research. While researching the literature it was found that Jouriles, Bourg, and Farris (1991) conducted a study which proved violent marital events where school-age children were involved was stronger in lower SES families than was found in higher SES families; however, literature is lacking if middle and upper class families meet this conclusion.

Studies on marital conflict effect on children shows a blend of both experimental and non-experimental design (El-Sheikh et al., 2008; Kuoros, Merrilees, & Cummings, 2008; Wymbs, 2008) providing evidence of suitability of the design in response to the research question. These studies provide a background to conducting the present study as they show many married couples have some form of aggression as a couple and expose their child to the conflict at home. Research estimating the reaction of children to the parent conflict focuses mainly on children's emotional behavior and inter-parent physical aggression rather than verbal aggression. Similar to the current study, the limiting factor for the studies is that participants need to have experience with parental conflict with children. Those studies focusing on adult's experiences identify that participants suffered some negative or positive effect from their childhood experiences.

The process of the study's sampling was non-random, which provided an opportunity to include participants who met the target for the study. Using a non-random sampling method has disadvantages for the study in that it creates a possibility for bias as the researcher looks for a target group of people (Chow, Wang, & Shao, 2008). For this study, non-random sampling presents the most ideal form of sampling because the focus is on having a select group of people who can adequately respond to the survey questions. For example, the qualifying criterion was for the participant to have witnessed verbal marital conflict as a child. Non-randomization of the sampling process increases the possibility of selecting people with such experiences and avoiding incomplete questionnaires.

The target sample size was 66 participants to be contacted through a survey company called SurveyGizmo. The sample was convenient in that qualifications were met through a set criterion. Participants needed to have witnessed verbal marital conflict as children to qualify for the study. The survey company was able to identify a sample based on the information provided, specifically the need for verbal marital conflict in childhood. Participants received an e-mail providing the particulars of the survey and asking them about their interest to participate if they qualify. Willing participants followed a link to the site for the survey where they received more information in the consent form provided. Participants gave electronic consent to participate or reject to participate by clicking their option of choice. The sampling occurred once with the survey company e-mailing invitations to 100 potential participants, and the sample was comprised of those persons who responded to the invitation.

The study population included men and women age 21 years and older. The expectation was to have people with varying demographic attributes such as their ethnicity, marital status, marital status of parents, number of children, and different employment capacities and industries. The demographic section of the survey had a comprehensive outlook on the participants' demographic attributes. The needed sample for the study was 66 participants, but the researcher requested for a contact of 100 potential participants. The reason for taking a large margin is to allow for incomplete questionnaires, and those participants that may not follow the link to complete the study. Achieving a 66% response rate will be sufficient for responding to the study. The appropriate number of participants was determined by using the 50+8(K) formula (Capella University, 2011), "K" being the number of variables or 2 (witnessing verbal marital conflict as a child and adult behavioral responses of anger. The total should therefore be at least 66 participants. However, due to potential uncompleted surveys, the sample size was 100. From this number, the researcher expected a 95% confidence level, on the possibility of rejecting the null hypothesis. The rejection is possible if the $p$ value is less than 0.05 (Borden & Abbott, 2011) after analysis of the data using SPSS (Statistical Package of Social Sciences).

## Procedures

The method of data collection was a web-based questionnaire. The web-based (online) questionnaire is largely replacing the paper and pen questionnaires, especially in the study of large populations. The reason is that it offers better probability of reaching large audiences with less large implications compared to the pen and paper questionnaires (van Gelder, Bretveld, & Roeleveld, 2010). Online questionnaires also provide the benefit of removing geographical and temporal boundaries (Howard, 2010). This makes it possible to recruit people from different geographical regions, and they can respond to the questionnaire at their convenience removing the need to adhere to time set by the research. However, the researcher set a time for the completion of the data collection, nullifying any questionnaires completed past that period.

The choice of a web-based questionnaire for this study was its settings, where it is possible to incorporate a requirement for participants to respond to all questions and move to the next based on their answer (Lumsden, 2007). For example, questions with compulsory responses have a setting where it is impossible for the respondent to move to the next question until they answer the present one. A concern in this regard is that such a setting forces respondents to select an option even when they would opt to forgo the question. The participants as noted in the consent form retain the right to withdraw from the study at any point by ending the interview. It was mandatory that each participant had to read a consent form and by clicking the option button to participate, the person would become a willing participant and agreed to take part in the study. Those that clicked the option button not to participate received a thank you message for considering to take part.

The researcher's e-mail address can be found on the consent form for the participants who are interested in requesting the results of the study. If participants feel the need to receive counseling after participating in the survey, the consent form had a toll free number for local area counseling referrals and a toll free number for emotional crisis support.

An online questionnaire has disadvantages that limit its effectiveness as a data collection tool. One disadvantage notable for this study is sampling issues, which reflects the challenge noted in non-experimental design. The researcher usually depends on the discretion of the participant to provide information qualifying them for the study but may not be able to verify that information (Bryman, 2012; Wright, 2005). Using an online company with registered members helps promote some degree of accuracy in the targeted population, but the researcher may not have the guarantee of reported characteristics if it was self-reported.

The researcher chose to use a web-based questionnaire because of available online research companies that make it easier to identify a sample and receive responses within an approximated timeframe. The selected survey company was SurveyGizmo. Using a survey company increases the possibility of having the questionnaires completed. Howard (2010) noted that evidence exists that web-based questionnaires are having a larger response rate compared to paper-based surveys.

SurveyGizmo is a software company that offers its customers access to a data collection tool within different pricing plans. It provides an easy distribution approach through e-mail invitations and social media platforms such as Twitter and Facebook (SurveyGizmo, 2014). A researcher can embed their survey through the company's website as a link. This study will use the e-mail option rather than sending a link to social media sites.

The procedure for collecting data involved purchasing a plan from SurveyGizmo and then uploading the questions based on the provided software development. Using SurveyGizmo it was possible to construct the questionnaire as both open and closed-ended questions. The questionnaire for this study had closed-ended questions. After uploading the questionnaire, the researcher chose the e-mail option, in which the company will send out an invitation to participate and an explanation of what the survey entailed. The invitation indicated the purpose of the survey, expectations of the researcher and participants, address confidentiality, time factor, and ensured the potential participants were aware participation was voluntary. From the invitation, participants who agreed to participate followed the link provided to be able to answer the questions. Prior to beginning the questionnaire, each participant had to show acceptance to participate by clicking on an option saying, "Yes, I choose to participate." Minimum age for participation is 21 years old, meaning that even if a participant indicates their willingness to participate they will need to pass the second question on age. The question is open. Persons younger than 21 years old received a thank you note and an indication that they do not qualify for the study.

Another advantage of using SurveyGizmo is that the company sends the data collected to the researcher in the form of an SPSS file for easier analysis. However, the researcher can access the raw questionnaires if need be, even though the file received has all the responses as they came into the system.

## Instruments

Surveys allow the researcher to build on existing tools if one so chooses instead of building a new tool. The form of survey used in this study was a self-completion questionnaire. Self-administration removes the need for the researcher to follow each participant to complete the tool (Amedeo, Golledge, & Stimson, 2012). The respondents attained the questionnaire online and submitted it online, making the process cheap and time effective as it does not require the researcher and respondent to plan on meetings, mail surveys or create flyers. The survey questionnaire had a combination of the Novaco Anger Scale (NAS; Novaco, 1994, 2003) and the Children's Perception of Interparental Conflict Scale (CPIC; Grych et al., 1992). The tools required participants to complete a demographic section asking about their area of residence, age, gender, ethnic background, their marital status and that of their parents. Participants completed both surveys fully.

The first part of the questionnaire was the consent form explaining the purpose of the study. It indicated what the researcher wanted to find out about adults exposed to verbal marital conflict as children and their anger response as an adult. The consent form include the targeted sample, age limitation, and benefits. The researcher noted that the participants should not expect any financial compensation for participating, and that the researcher was also not receiving funding to conduct the study. The results would be of use in creating solutions for others exposed to verbal marital conflict but may not benefit the participant directly. Considering the questionnaire required participants to remember times that could have been traumatic, the consent form provided a toll free number for emotional support incase participants felt they would require counseling after the study.

The consent form assured participants of confidentiality, but noted the challenge of internet risks including hacking. Confidentiality may also not apply in cases of noted abuse and planned harm to one's self or others.

The questionnaire contained closed ended questions. For example, a question in the CPIC scale (Grych et al., 1992) required participants to select one of five answer options for such a statement mentioning if they ever saw their parents disagreeing. The possible responses included: almost never, rarely, occasionally, often, and almost always. A scale with options such as these is considered a Likert scale. Another example of a closed ended question was to indicate the years one has been married or the state the participant lived. One section of the questionnaire was the demographic survey containing information on gender, ethnic background, education, marital status of parents, guardianship as a child, employment, and family background. The remaining section after the demographic survey was the NAS (Novaco, 1994, 2003) and the CPIC (Grych et al., 1992) scales.

**The Novaco Anger Scale**

The Novaco Anger Scale (NAS; Novaco, 1994, 2003) is an ordinal scale with three points, "Never true, sometimes true, and always true." The scale developed in 1994 from the work of Novaco (1976) on the model of anger management was modified in 2003 (Jones, Thomas-Peter, & Gangstad, 2003). There are four subscales: cognitive, arousal, behavioral, and anger regulation. It has an additional section called the Provocation Inventory (PI) that test the kind of situations leading to anger including: disrespect, unfairness, frustration, annoyance by others, and irritations. The researcher has a choice to administer the NAS (NAS; Novaco, 1994, 2003) together with the

Provocation Inventory (PI) or separately. The choice depends on whether the researcher feels the respondent may fail to complete the entire questionnaire because of fatigue or if the PI scale is necessary for the research. The focus of the study also gives the researcher liberty to choose one part of the scale.

The usefulness of the tool in measurement of anger is its internal consistency with researchers testing its value concluding that it was a valuable tool for assessment of anger in tested groups (Culhane & Morera, 2010; Hornsveld & Kraaimaat, 2011). The scale has 60 items that a respondent can complete in 15 minutes with focus being on how an individual responds to anger or their experiences with anger. For this study, the respondents will have to respond to the entire NAS (Novaco, 1994, 2003) to avoid participation manipulation, although the part pertinent to this study is the behavior subscale. Its original reliability test, the internal reliability was .94 for the NAS (Novaco, 1994, 2003) and .95 for the Provocation Inventory (Novaco, n. d.). The NAS (Novaco, 1994, 2003) subscale reliability ranges from .76 to .89. The alpha for the NAS (Novaco, 1994, 2003) behavior subscale is .89. Regarding validity of the scale, initial tests noted that the scale showed significant correlations in expected variables. Based on the tests for reliability and validity, the researcher expects the study will show expected outcomes.

**The Children's Perception of Interparental Conflict Scale**

The CPIC (Grych et al., 1992) scale comes from the work of Grych, Seid, and Fincham (1992) that assessed marital conflict from the perspective of a child. The development of the CPIC (Grych et al., 1992) was to test children on different perspectives especially on the properties of conflict, perceived threat, and self-blame (Bickham & Fiese, 1997; Moura, Santos, Rocha, & Matos, 2010). The scale has five points "almost never true, rarely true, occasionally true, often true, and always true." In its maiden use, the CPIC scale (Grych et al., 1992) showed acceptable levels of internal consistency within the three subscales (Grych et al., 1992). The findings further showed significant relations between the reports of conflict and child assessment measurement for the conflict properties subscale. The other two scales also showed significant correlation. The reliability range was between .80 and .89 (Bickham & Fiese, 1997). The scale contains 49 statements. The participants will respond to all 49 statements; however, there are two questions pertaining to physical violence which will not be used in the data analysis. Considering the tool has confirmed reliability and validity tests, the researcher expects it to provide empirical evidence to nullify the null hypothesis resulting in a significant relationship between children witnessing verbal marital conflict and its effect on adulthood anger responses.

## Research Questions and Hypothesis

The research question explored in this study is: What is the relationship between witnessing verbal marital conflict as a child and the behavior of anger responses as an adult?

*Ho:* The null hypothesis for this study is: There is no significant relationship between witnessing verbal marital conflict as a child and the behavior of anger responses as an adult.

*H:* The alternative hypothesis for this study is: There is a significant relationship between witnessing verbal marital conflict as a child and the behavior of anger responses as an adult.

## Data Analysis

The process of the data analysis began with retrieval of the completed questionnaires from SurveyGizmo. The expectation was to have at least 95% of the questionnaire responses at the close of the survey. The data from SurveyGizmo was in SPSS (Statistical Package of Social Sciences), which is the statistical software used for the data analysis. The reason for choosing SPSS is so the researcher could conduct a correlation analysis. A Spearman's Rank Order Correlation was performed through SPSS 18.0. The software has other advantages such as creation of tables and graphs through determining the frequency distribution of the data collected and making comparisons between variables (Carver & Nash, 2011). SPSS provides an adequate software for data analysis. Noted, the researcher does not expect to manually enter the data into the software because the data report can export from SurveyGizmo to the SPSS software.

During the data analysis process all the information collected was stored in a computer protected with a password to safeguard the information. The researcher also had a password for access of SurveyGizmo data for added protection of the information in case of any problems with the computer. During the analysis process, the researcher continually uploaded the information as a report through SurveyGizmo to ensure the information was available. This ensured easy retrieval in case of data corruption such as through a virus or loss of computer. At completion of the data analysis, the researcher will delete the information saved on the computer, but retain the information online through reports. This will mean the researcher could retrieve the information later if needed. Safeguarding the information is important until the research process including the completion of the report is complete.

Participants may request a copy of the findings by sending an e-mailed request to the researcher's e-mail address found on the consent form. Confirmation will ensure the researcher does not release the analyzed results to persons not involved in the process or those without any significant interest in the findings such as psychology professionals. The academia will also have access to the completed report as necessary.

**Ethical Considerations**

This study was approved by Capella University's Institutional Review Board (IRB), which ensured that there was no violation of the participants' human rights (2012). As the research involved psychological aspects such as people remembering their past, the participants could need psychological intervention in case the process of remembering causes psychological trauma. The researcher does not intend any harm from conducting the study, but recognizes the possibility. The consent form the participants electronically sign noted the possibility of this occurring and advised participants to seek psychiatric attention if it becomes necessary. As noted, taking the survey was at the discretion of the participant and the researcher will not accept liability for any occurrences that require medical attention. The consent form indicated the need for the participants to be sure they were able to handle any arising psychological concerns prior to beginning the study.

Another consideration in the research was that confidentiality is most often the primary focus of ethical concern in survey research. Confidentiality is an assurance to the participants that the researcher will safeguard their information and can only release it to authorized persons. The researcher assured the participants from the beginning of observing confidentiality as indicated in the consent form explaining the purpose of the study. However, assurances of privacy in the study have limits where the researcher feels that the participant may or may have caused him/herself harm or to another person. In such a case, the rights to confidentiality are waived. Generally, the researcher has safeguarded the information provided throughout the survey. The information can however be accessible to supervisors or other authorized persons if necessary.

Connected to confidentiality is the issue of anonymity. The researcher advised all participants not to provide any personal information that someone else could use to identify them. Agreeably, this study required the participant to provide some personal information such as age, marital status, employment, schooling, and their parent's marital status in the demographic questions. Such information is not personally identifying compared to a combination of factors such as date of birth and social security number. The survey does not expect the participants to provide such information, but focused on their experiences and perceptions of anger responses and verbal marital conflict.

Another ethical consideration was the informed consent form denoting the participant freely agreeing to take part in the study after receiving information on the nature of the study (Kimmel, 2007). The participants received a consent form informing them of the expectations of the research, the role of the participants, and benefits of the study. From the consent form, the participants are aware that the study will not give them any tangible benefits. At the end of reading the consent form, the participants will electronically agree or disagree to participate in the study. Those who selected *yes* by indication showed they understood the consent and were willing to take part in the study within the set parameters.

In order to safeguard the information on the computer, all the information collected was protected with a password. In addition, SurveyGizmo was also password protected. All the research data on the computer would be deleted at the conclusion of the study, but would still be available online through reports.

Conducting a web-based survey raises additional concerns on how to ensure the instrument reaches the expected persons and they respond to the questionnaire once. The researcher took the necessary steps to ensure the questionnaire could only be completed once by each participant. SurveyGizmo provides a filter ensuring only one response per registered member. The participants received the invitation to take the survey from their e-mail and followed a link to the site, this could act as a deterrence to responding numerous times.

**Expected Findings**

The expectation of this research was to disprove the null hypothesis by showing that witnessing verbal marital conflict as a child affects behavioral anger responses in adulthood. Through calculation of correlation, the research intended to demonstrate that adults exposed to verbal marital conflict in childhood have a greater likelihood of responding in anger compared to those exposed to mild or low verbal marital conflict. The study used findings from the Novaco Anger Scale (NAS; 1994, 2003) and the Children Perception of Interparental Conflict Scale (CPIC; Grych et al., 1992). The first scale provided an indicator for anger responses, and the latter scale showed the relationship in the conflict. An element to note is that not all children exposed to verbal marital conflict will have challenges dealing with anger in adulthood, considering each child formulates a coping model that suits their capabilities. However, some children may carry the emotional wounds suffered in childhood to their adulthood forming a background for anger response to exposed stimuli. The expectation was that for some children the exposure to anger will have a destructive impact on their emotional development and social functioning; as a result, affecting their lifestyle and interaction with others.

Possible findings will be that the participants will provide evidence of the relationship between behavior anger responses as adults, which relates to exposure to verbal marital conflict as children. The study will provide empirical evidence disproving the null hypothesis and that will contribute to the identified research gap on the impact of witnessing verbal marital conflict.

## Summary

This chapter outlined the data collection method for the current study. The study was quantitative with an expected sample of 66 participants. The criteria for the study was that the participants must have witnessed verbal marital conflict as a child. The participants granted permission to take part in the study by acceptance of the consent form provided with the survey, and indicated they had experienced verbal marital conflict. The study used SurveyGizmo, an online survey company for recruitment of participants. The participants received an e-mailed questionnaire from the survey company. The questionnaire consisted of a demographic section, the NAS (Novaco; 1994, 2003) and the CPIC (Grych et al., 1992). The following chapter presents the findings of the survey.

# CHAPTER 4. DATA COLLECTION AND ANALYSIS

## Introduction

The purpose of this chapter is to present the data collected and analyzed from the survey. The chapter provides an analysis based on the three parts of the questionnaire: the demographic section, the Novaco Anger Scale (NAS; 1994, 2003), and the Children's Perception of Interparental Conflict Scale (CPIC; Grych, et al., 1992). It begins with a recap on the study process by describing the sampling and then the response rate, followed by the demographic details of the sample, results of the CPIC (Grych, et al., 1992), and then results of the NAS (Novaco; 1994, 2003). The chapter includes an analysis of whether the results show a correlation between witnessing verbal marital conflict as a child with anger responses as an adult.

## Description of the Sample

The sampling procedure was non-random and conducted using SurveyGizmo, an online company. The qualification for participation was having witnessed verbal marital conflict as a child and be 21 years of age and older. Through SurveyGizmo, the participants received an e-mail providing details of the survey and asking for their participation. The target for this study was to identify 66 participants who could respond to the surveys. However, due to potential uncompleted surveys, the sample size was 100. The response rate was 100 percent, as the 100 persons targeted in the sampling responded fully to the questionnaire. The 100 counted were those who selected "Yes, I will participate." The responses came in within the established timeframe; therefore, the researcher did not need to disqualify any responses for lateness. As set within the questionnaire, the participants were not able to overlook any questions because each participant had to answer the previous question to proceed to the next. The researcher did not attain incomplete questionnaires. The full sample of 100 was therefore admissible for the study.

The data analysis was through SPSS (Statistical Package for Social Studies). The data analysis began by exploration of the demographic aspects of the questionnaires and then finding correlations between the targeted items in the NAS (Novaco, 1994, 2003) and the CPIC (Grych et al., 1992) scales.

**Demographics**

The target age group for the study were individuals aged 21 years old and older. Those responding to the study were from 22 years old to 69 years old. The majority of the participants were aged between 36 to 40 years old ($n = 23$) followed by 31 to 35 years old ($n = 18$) and then by 46 to 50 years old ($n = 16$). Table 1 provides the frequency distribution per age group based on the current study and a comparison to the U.S. Census data (2012) consisting of the ages and percentages which make up the U.S. population. The age representation for the study was done in similar fashion to that of the census which requires participants to indicate age and date of birth. The present study required the age, and from this the researcher grouped the respondents. The census grouping has both wide margins and margins of five years such as 20-24 years (Howden & Meyer, 2011), which was the margin of choice in the current study as it shows greater representation of the participants' age. Based on U.S. Census data (2012) ages 21-44 makes up a population percentage of 31.9. Ages 45-64 make up 26.5% and ages 65 years and over totals 13.4%.

Table 1
*Age Representation of Participants*

| Age | Frequency/Percentage | U.S. Census Percentage |
|---|---|---|
| 20-24 | 2 | 7.1 |
| 25-29 | 2 | 6.8 |
| 30-34 | 15 | 6.6 |
| 35-39 | 21 | 6.2 |
| 40-44 | 17 | 6.7 |
| 45-49 | 15 | 7 |
| 50-54 | 12 | 7.2 |
| 55-59 | 7 | 6.6 |
| 60-64 | 7 | 5.7 |
| 65-69 | 2 | 4.4 |

All the participants (100%) indicated that they had experienced verbal marital conflict between their parents. The indicators for marital conflict as provided in the explanation to participants where situations characterized by significant levels of verbal conflict, distrust, poor communication, anger, and cooperation such as in parenting, and an ongoing harmful attitude toward one's partner (McIntosh, 2010). The definition also noted that verbal marital conflict did not include physical violence.

Table 2
*Gender Representation*

| Gender | Percentage | U.S. Census Percentage |
|---|---|---|
| Male | 82 | 49.2 |
| Female | 18 | 50.8 |
| Total | 100 | 100 |

The female participants represented 82% ($n = 82$) of the participants, with the male participants representing 18%. The item on gender is representative of the national census format which requests participants to indicate whether they are male of female without any other characterization.

Table 3
*Ethnic Representation*

| Race | Percentage | U. S. Census Percentage |
|---|---|---|
| White | 33 | 77.9 |
| African American/Black | 60 | 13.1 |
| American Indian | 2 | 1.2 |
| Asian | 1 | 5.1 |
| Native Hawaiian and Other Pacific Islander | 0 | 0.2 |
| Two or More Races | 0 | 2.4 |

The ethnic/racial representation showed that the majority of participants as featured on Table 3 were African American or Black ($n = 60$).

The Native Hawaii/Pacific Islander category did not have any representation. American Indian or Alaska Native were represented by 2 participants, while Asian, and others were represented by 1 and 4 participants, respectively. Those that chose *other* explained their ethnic or racial background as Latino, Hispanic and mixed race. The White category was the second highest ($n = 33$) represented following the African American category. Within the racial background, participants were asked to indicate their Hispanic background with the findings shown in Table 4. U.S. Census data (2012) pertaining to the ethnic population can also be found on tables 3 and 4.

Table 4
*Hispanic Origin of Participants*

| Race | Percentage | U. S. Census Percentage |
|---|---|---|
| Hispanic or Latino | 3 | 16.9 |
| White alone, Black alone, not Hispanic or Latino | 93 | 63 |
| Mexican, Mexican American, or Chicano | 1 | 0.0 |
| Puerto Rican | 2 | 0.0 |
| Cuban | 1 | 0.0 |

It was found that the majority of the participants were not of Hispanic origin and this was consistent with the racial/ethnic findings where the majority were African American or Black, or White ($n = 93$). Table 4 provides a breakdown of the specific Hispanic Origin of any participant. The reason for considering the Hispanic and non-Hispanic origins is to align to the national census that classifies between as either Hispanic in origin or non-Hispanic in origin (U.S. Census Bureau, 2012). The categories provided through the Census are White alone, mixed race, Black/African American alone, American Indian and Alaska Native alone, Asian, and Native Hawaiian and other Pacific Islander alone (U.S. Census Bureau, 2012). The study included the Cuban classification due to researcher interactions with persons who classified themselves as such.

Table 5
*Marital Status of the Parents*

| Marital Status | Percentage |
| --- | --- |
| Divorced parents | 39 |
| Still married parents | 61 |

Many of the participants indicated that their parents were married ($n = 89$), while 11 noted that their parents did not marry. Marriage and divorce is part of the household measurement in the national census along with separated, never married and with a category of widowhood (Elliot & Simmons, 2011), but only the first two categories were required for this study.

Table 6
*Raised By a Parent or Parental Figure*

| | Percentage |
| --- | --- |
| Two parents | 59 |
| One parent | 17 |
| One parental figure | 2 |
| Two parental figures | 8 |
| One parent and one parental figure | 14 |

Participants were required to state whether a parent or parental figure raised them. Many of the participants indicated both parents raised them ($n = 59$) as shown on Table 6 above. The findings indicated that many of the participants had at least a parent raise them ($n = 76$), while others were raised by a single parent ($n = 17$). Fourteen participants indicated that they were raised by a parent with another parental figure. The participants raised by two parents unanimously indicated that they were raised by a male and female parent. The majority of participants raised by a single parent were the female parent ($n = 16$) with one raised by the male parent. Those raised by a parental figure had equal representation with one male and one female. Participants raised by two parental figures chose the option that these were parents comprised of one male and one female couple(s). For those raised by one parent and one parental figure, the majority ($n = 13$) noted the parent was female and the parental figure was male, with one participant noting both the parent and parental figure were female. However, all the participants ($n = 100$) noted they were not raised in a home with same sex partners.

## Summary of Results

The results of the study showed that there is no statistical significant relationship between experiencing verbal marital conflict as a child and the behavioral anger response as an adult. The Spearman correlation showed no significant relationship with a correlation coefficient of $r^2 = 0.101$.

The research question answered was: What is the relationship between witnessing verbal marital conflict as a child and the behavior of anger responses as an adult. The study tested various elements to show exposure to verbal marital conflict as a child and others testing the responses the exposed child developed into adulthood. Many participants ($n = 24$) noted that they *almost never* saw their parents arguing, and those that argued mainly worked out their differences when they occurred based on the options *occasionally true* ($n = 31$), *often true* ($n = 24$), *almost always true* ($n = 14$). Further on parents behavior, the participants indicated that their parents became very angry after arguing based on options *occasionally true* (*n* = 25), *often true* (*n* = 26), *almost always true* (*n* = 29). Many of the participants indicated that as children they did not feel caught in the middle of the arguments of their parents with 24 participants choosing *almost never true* and 25 choosing *rarely true*. To determine the child's response to the interparental conflict, the participants indicated how they felt about their parent's verbal marital conflict. Many felt they were to blame for the conflict (*n* = 42) choosing *almost always true* and 27 choosing *often true*.

To test behavioral anger responses as a child, the tools reflected the behavior of participants as adults. The findings showed that many of the participants felt their temper was not quick and hot (*n* = 53) and those indicating they had a temper *sometimes* (*n* = 40). In addition, the majority of the participants (*n* = 68) agreed that it was *sometimes true* that they yelled back when yelled at while 50 of the participants agreed to responding with roughness when provoked. A considerable number of participants (*n* = 68) indicated that it was *never true* in response to the question indicating that they felt like smashing things. Many of the participants (*n* = 76) indicated that if someone hit them they would hit back.

Based on the behavioral findings and the correlation, the findings approved the null hypothesis centrally to the research expectations. Through Spearman's Rank Order one tailed correlation coefficient, the results showed $r^2 = 0.101$ with the significance being $p = 0.159$. The expectation of the study was $p < 0.05$ which would prove the alternative hypothesis, but instead it proved the null hypothesis which rejected the alternative hypothesis. The study showed that there was no significance relationship between witnessing verbal marital conflict as a child and the behavior of anger responses as an adult.

## Details of the Analysis and Results

The following documentation will show the specific analysis of data collection based on the questions. The first section will be the demographics of the participants, followed by the CPIC (Grych et al., 1992) and NAS (Novaco; 1994, 2003) findings. The section will conclude with a discussion of the disproved findings of the study's hypothesis.

## Children's Perception of Their Parents Conflict

This section assessed the participants' perception of verbal conflicts witnessed between parents. To establish witnessing of verbal marital conflict, participants responded to whether they ever saw their parents arguing. Table 7 shows the responses, with 1 being *almost never true*, 2 was *rarely true*, 3 was *occasionally true*, 4 was *often true* and 5 was *almost always true*. The same scale replicates with the rest of the items in this section.

Table 7
*Witnessing Parental Arguments*

|  | Frequency | Percentage |
|---|---|---|
| Almost never true | 24 | 24 |
| Rarely true | 25 | 25 |
| Occasionally true | 25 | 25 |
| Often true | 18 | 18 |
| Almost always true | 8 | 8 |

The majority of the participants indicated at some point in time they have seen their parents arguing, with eight participants indicating they *almost always* saw parents having an argument. Eighteen participants chose *often true*, while many were in the third and fourth categories choosing *occasionally true* ($n = 25$) and *rarely true* ($n = 25$). Twenty four percent of participants chose *almost never true* to seeing their parents arguing, which may indicate some participant confusion as witnessing such arguing was a criteria for participation in the study. The participants noted that many of the parents worked out their differences following the argument. There were those that chose *almost always true* ($n = 14$), while 24 chose *often true*, 31 chose *occasionally true*, 18 chose *rarely true*, and 13 chose *almost never true*. The participants also noted their parents' behavior when they were arguing, with the indicator being on whether the parents became mad or very angry.

The findings showed that the majority of participants ($n = 29$) selected *almost always true* in response to the question about their parents being very angry following an argument, while 26 indicated *often true,* 25 responded with *occasionally true,* 12 choosing *rarely true*, and eight choosing *almost never true*.

**Behavioral Anger Response**

The NAS (Novaco; 1994, 2003) items used in the analysis are those on behavioral anger response to stimuli. One item was on whether their temper was quick and hot. The participants were selecting between *never true, sometimes true*, and *always true* in a Likert scale of three elements which remain standard for the rest of the section on anger response. The majority of the participants ($n = 53$) indicated it was not true that their anger was quick and hot, while 40 participants indicated to sometimes having a quick and hot temper. Only seven participants agreed that their temper was always quick and hot.

Another item was about yelling back when someone yelled at the participant. The majority of participants ($n = 68$) noted this was *sometimes true* at, while 21 participants stated that it was not true they yelled back and 11 participants agreed to *always* yelling back. With regards to being rough with people that bothered the participants, the emerging feeling was that many chose ($n = 50$) the option sometimes responded in roughness, while 44 participants stated this was *never true* for them. Six of the participants indicated this was *always true* for them.

The participants further indicated whether they felt like smashing things. The response was mainly that this was *never true* ($n = 68$), with 30 participants agreeing to sometimes feeling like smashing things, and two participants noting the element was *always true* for them. Another element was participants reacting first when someone bothers them and then thinking about it later. Many of the participants said this was not true ($n = 55$). However, 44 participants felt this was *sometimes true* w, and one participant feeling this was always the case. The responses of the participants, pertaining to the item associated with their angry was consistent with their response on temper. For example, while 53 participants indicated it was not true their temper was quick and hot, 65 participants noted that it was not true they flew of the handle unknowingly when angry. Another consistency noted was on items of taking out anger on someone else and knocking people around, with 78 and 77 participants, respectively, indicating this was *never true*.

**Clinical Relevance**

The scores of the CPIC (Grych et al., 1992) and NAS (Novaco, 1994, 2003) provide an indication into the clinical relevance of the findings. Based on a rating scale identified in other studies, it was possible to assess if the findings showed an indicator on clinically significant scores (Nikolas et al., 2012; Yip et al., 2012). The considerations for the CPIC (Grych et al., 1992) were the scores that showed low, moderate, and high scores based on a range of 47 to 235 from the lowest to the highest. The lower range was between 47 and 109, the moderate scale was 110 to 172, and 173 – 253 for high scores. The higher score would show clinical significance could be the need for an intervention. The average for the scores was 124.36 with a 20.1286 standard deviation. Table 8 shows the number of participants relative to the range.

Table 8
*Total Scores for CPIC*

| Range | Percentage |
| --- | --- |
| 47 - 109 | 27 |
| 110 – 172 | 72 |
| 173 -235 | 1 |

The findings showed that majority of the participants score was average falling on the moderate position. One person qualified for clinical intervention having scored above 173. The minimum score was to be 47 with a maximum of 235.

Scores on the NAS (Novaco, 1994, 2003) range from 16 to 48. Similar to the CPIC (Grych et al., 1992), the test was for clinical relevance with the higher end scores indicating a need for clinical interventions. Pertaining to the findings shown on Table 9, two participants scored within the high level while the others remained in the moderate category. The average score was 24.85 with a standard deviation of 4.468.

Table 9
*NAS Clinical Relevance Test*

| Range | Percentage |
|---|---|
| 16 – 26 | 65 |
| 27 – 37 | 33 |
| 38 – 48 | 2 |

Based on the clinical test, witnessing verbal marital conflict does not seem to be an indicator for a clinically significant anger response that would need clinical intervention; however, only 1% and 2% of the participants in the CPIC (Grych et al., 1992) and NAS (Novaco, 1994, 2003), respectively, show a need for an intervention.

**Relationship Between Witnessing Verbal Marital Conflict and Anger Response**

The calculation for finding the correlation between witnessing verbal marital conflict as a child and the behavior of anger responses as an adult sought to show whether the findings would feature a significant impact evident with $p < 0.05$ (Borden & Abbott, 2011). Using Spearman one-tailed correlation coefficient resulted with an $r^2 = 0.101$ that the findings were not significant at the 0.05 level ($p = 0.159$).

Based on the findings, there was no significant relationship between witnessing verbal marital conflict as a child, as measured by the CPIC, and the behavior of anger responses as an adult, as measured by the NAS behavior subscale. The results showed mixed anger reactions. For example, participants indicated to sometimes yelling at people that yell at them, as noted by 68 of the participants, while 50 participants believed in roughing up others. Similarly the participants had instances of non-response behavior where they would not move into violence based on the actions of another person; therefore based on the data, it seems there may be a possibility their actions in volatile situations may not relate directly to childhood experiences.

## Conclusion

The findings indicated in this section highlighted the behavioral anger responses of people who witnessed verbal conflicts growing up. All the participants implied to having been witnesses to verbal marital conflicts; however, it seems some participants may have misunderstood the meaning of "witnessing" the conflicts. The 24 participants who initially consented to the study to witnessing verbal marital conflict responded as if it was never true that they witnessed their parents arguing or disagreeing, showing some confusion. Although, the magnitude of the conflict differed as noted when participants were responding to whether they saw their parents arguing or disagreeing, and parents being able to resolve their differences. The reactions further differed as seen with some children blaming themselves for their parents' actions or feeling they were to blame for the conflict. The next section provides an analysis of the findings and compares the current results to those noted in literature about how verbal marital conflict affects children. The chapter further offers conclusions of the study and recommendations focusing on the practice of counseling and future research.

# CHAPTER 5. RESULTS, CONCLUSIONS, AND RECOMMENDATIONS

## Introduction

The purpose of the study was to explore the relationship between witnessing verbal marital conflict as a child and the behavior of anger responses as an adult. The study used the Novaco Anger Scale (Novaco; NAS, 1994, 2003) and the Children's Perception of Interparental Conflict Scale (CPIC; Grych et al., 1992) to determine their response to anger. The findings as presented in the previous chapter showed that people have varying reactions when angered or confronted with angry situations. The following chapter explores the connection of the current findings with previous literature about anger responses and the impact of marital conflict on children. This chapter contains a summary of the findings and a discussion that compares and contrasts the findings of the current study to previous research. It provides supporting literature to the findings in cases where such support was not provided in the literature review and study background.

## Summary of the Results

The way a child learns how to handle conflict is first learned through observing the family in the household (Feldman, Mashalha, & Derdikman-Eiron, 2010). The purpose of this study was to analyze the social learning and emotional security of adults who witnessed verbal marital conflict as children. Based on the study, if the adults displayed an answer in the survey that their anger responses currently showed parallel relation to witnessing this conflict, then therapeutic designs and interventions would benefit the adult greatly.

The current study sought to examine if there was a relationship between witnessing verbal marital conflict as a child and the behavior of anger responses as an adult. The findings showed the feelings and responses of adults who experienced verbal conflicts between their parents as children had no significant relationship to their angered behavior in adulthood. The study design was a non-experimental, correlational design using two survey tools for the data collection. The survey tools formed a questionnaire defining verbal marital conflict and asking participants to reflect upon witnessing verbal marital conflict as a child and anger responses as an adult. The important aspect is recognizing that the couples raising the child produced some form of conflict witnessed by the child. The qualifying factor for participation in the study was that the participants must have been 21 years and older and witnessed verbal marital conflict as children although the magnitude of the conflict differed.

The null hypothesis was proven by showing that witnessing verbal marital conflict as a child did not affect anger responses in adulthood. The findings as shown in chapter 4, the calculation of correlation did not show a significant relationship between the two variables as the correlation coefficient $r^2 = 0.101$. This suggested that experiencing verbal conflict as a child as measured by the CPIC (Grych et al., 1992) was not significantly correlated with behavior anger responses in adulthood as measured by the NAS (Novaco, 1994, 2003). For a significant relationship to emerge between the dependent and independent variables the value of $p$ needed to be below 0.05. The Spearman's Rank Order 1-tailed relationship coefficient showed $p = 0.159$ which proved the null hypothesis. As shown in in chapter 4, the coefficient was higher than the set limit therefore confirming the null hypothesis. The conclusion of the study is that witnessing verbal conflict is not an indicator of how a person will respond to anger stimulus in adulthood. Being that more of the responses were on the middle level such as choosing *sometimes* rather than the extreme level on each survey is a good indication as to the relationship of witnessing verbal marital conflict and behavior responses in adulthood.

The findings showed that on many of the statements, the participants did not show behavior anger responses, which could have been a potential sign in having challenges in anger response as adults. For example, the statements on whether the participants had a hot temper, yelled back, smashed things when angered, or even reacted first without thinking, showed the participants opted for the average position. This means it was not true that they had a hot temper. The results indicated that the participants' anger responses were not challenged by experiencing verbal marital conflict as children.

The CPIC (Grych et al., 1992) provided a critical guide into how experiencing verbal marital conflict affected a child, but not how it impacted the behavior in adulthood. The NAS (Novaco, 1994, 2003) was to offer such insight but the suggestion seemed that the adults did not suffer unduly in anger response because of such exposure, hence the acceptance of the null hypothesis. Experiencing verbal marital conflict between parents did not mean a person would have excessive behavioral anger response as an adult.

The findings in this study did not align with previous research. The literature showed that exposure to parental verbal conflict as children may cause externalization and internalization behavior among children even as they grow into adulthood (El-Sheikh et al., 2009; Fosco & Grych, 2008; Obradovic, Bush, & Boyce, 2011). Such findings explained why people might react violently under little provocation. For example, a person may become violent even under minimum provocation, which is because they are defending themselves. Literature on externalization shows that children display emotional challenges and self-blame as part of eternalizing problems (El-Sheikh et al., 2013; Zarling et al., 2013). Suggested by such findings is that perception of threat links to maladjustment and the emotional reaction of children to threat and self-blame. The current study showed that children felt they were to blame for their parents conflict with $n = 27$ selecting *often true*, and $n = 47$ *almost always true*.

Previous research suggests that the problem with externalization was that children received poor socialization and poor management of conflicts, and they carry the same approach into their adulthood (Davies et al., 2012; Faircloth, 2012). This explains the reason some people have challenges in maintaining a good intimate relationship. The current research, however, presented a different outlook. While some participants showed poor responses such as in reaction to anger responses, a large portion of participants responded moderately. For example, many participants noted that when angry they did not hit others ($n = 81$), or slam things ($n = 68$). Other questions indicated that the participants may react angrily, for example, when asked if when provoked they fly off the handle without knowing, $n = 65$ stated it was *not true*, $n = 33$ stated it was *sometimes true*, and $n = 2$ indicated it was always true. The findings of this study showed mixed reactions in some areas, but mainly showed that exposure to anger was not a reason for angry responses.

**Conclusions on Impact of Marital Conflict on Children**

The literature review showed that couples often have conflicts as part of the marriage interaction (Cummings & Davies, 2011). The children may become exposed to the conflict not by intention of the couple but because they are part of the family. For some couples, they are able to address the conflict before it becomes a problem to the entire family or it breaks down communication between the couple. The literature review showed the importance of children being exposed to conflict resolution methods as part of the family unit, because the family is a socialization agent (Bern, 2013). Based on the socialization concept, the family can teach children how to react to situations of conflict, which can be negative or positive. This means that children who learn conflict resolution methods will likely adopt such methods when confronted with conflicts later (Grych & Fincham, 1990). Similarly, children that fail to learn conflict resolution techniques within the family will have challenges in resolving conflicts. Additionally, a positive home environment helps children to create healthy relationships later in life (Grych & Fincham, 1990). The techniques they adopt when forming relationships become instrumental to future relationships. The way parents manage conflicts has a greater likelihood of influencing how children adjust compared to the conflict itself. The outlook emerging from literature was that the effect of exposure to conflict between parents depended both upon the manner of expressing the conflict, management and resolution, and the extent children felt they were to blame for the conflict as well as perceived threat (Grych et al., 2003). This study showed that sometimes children felt at fault when their parents were engaged in a conflict, or felt caught in the middle and scared of the conflict. This could explain the reason marital conflict could be a source of anxiety for children exposed. However, this study noted that parents were able to resolve their conflicts in many instances suggesting conflict resolution development among the children.

Previous research has noted that exposure to marital conflict affects the development of children (Cui & Fincham, 2010; Davies et al., 2012; Fosco, et al., 2007; Laurent et al., 2008; Nicholas & Rasmussen, 2006; Pauli-Pott & Dieter, 2007; Sturge-

Apple et al., 2008). Based on the social emotional theory, children may become exposed to the conflicts creating doubts into their security (Singh, 2010). When parents argue, children feel threatened especially if the argument shows signs of escalation and the children could feel caught in the argument. Ideally, parents provide a safety net for their children, but exposure to conflict could fracture this safety. The literature review suggested that children exposed to parent conflict may adopt behaviors as defense mechanisms including siding with one parent (Cummings & Davies, 2010).

Previous literature highlighted the implications of discordant through non-violent conflict between parents; showing it had negative implications for the children, and showing a need for professionals and policy makers to stop identifying conflict between parents as simply violence being present or not (Cummings & Davies, 2010; Rhoades, 2008). Usually response to domestic conflict has been based on violent tendencies, which denies intervention to the emotional aspects arising from exposure to non-violent conflict (Rhoades, 2008). Practitioners need to consider that conflicts between parents include various factors, both emotional and physical, and could range from aggressive silence to violent behavior.

Based on previous literature the impact of marital conflict can cause negative effect in children whether the hostility was overt or covert (Amato, 2001). This means that parents whose conflict is mainly marked by emotional withdrawal has the capacity to affect the emotional and behavioral development of their children within a similar strength to those with poor but overt conflicts. Parents may claim that their relationship did not have poor interaction or they did not expose their conflict to their children so no poor impact should be found in their environment. The aspect of silent fighting in covert conflict will have considerable implications on the children affecting their ability to form lasting relationships (Amato, 2001).

A large number of literature supports the possibility of conflict causing developmental challenges in children and poor academic achievement (Cavanagh & Huston 2006; Cavanagh, Schiller, & Riegle-Crumb 2006; Fomby & Cherlin 2007; Heard 2007a; Osborne & McLanahan 2007). This impact results from the socialization aspect of families as arising conflict affects the character of children and their quality of behavior (Heard 2007b; Heaton & Forste 2007). Based on the social learning theory (SLT), families form a system that teach children how to function in society (Bandura, 1969). Conflict can cause disruptions to this system and its functionality with the possibility of causing long-term problems in behavioral development in children. This occurs for family with biological parents and those with parental figures. Children exposed to parental conflict can also cause a stressful environment that can have long term implications on the health and performance of a child.

The literature available on the effect of parental conflict on children's anger management suggest that children may develop models of anger and conflict resolution based on the models adopted by their parents (DeBaryshe & Fryxell, 2013). By observing how their parents deal with anger, children form mental images on response to aggression, with researchers finding significant correlation between exposure and attitude towards anger and anger regulation (Kinsfogel & Grych, 2004). The current study; however, showed that exposure to parental conflict did not propose the child would have challenges with anger regulation as an adult. The findings showed that many of the participants did not have a quick temper. Although some participants indicated to having a quick temper ($n = 7$) this did not qualify as a significant number. The participants noted that they sometimes had a quick temper.

At this time, the literature in this area published in the last five years is lacking, and older works of literature in this area pertaining to anger response in connection to verbal marital conflict does not provide an adequate relationship between the two subjects at hand.

## Discussion of the Results

This study responded to the identified problem of whether experiencing verbal marital conflict affected a person into adulthood. During the literature review, it was clear that exposure to marital conflict affected children in emotional development and academic outcome (Davies & Cummings, 1994). The impact is evident through internalizing and externalizing behaviors (Beuhler, et al., 2007; Davies & Cummings, 1998). Lacking in literature was however the impact of exposure to verbal conflict and the way such exposure affected a person as an adult. The study sought to understand if such exposure affected the way a person responded to anger provocation. The basis of the study was that although a child may not be an active participant in the conflict, he or she could hear the parents arguing or see the outcome and this could have a bearing on their development. Possible consequences were in learning how to interact with others and resolve conflicts. The family is a socialization unit from where children understand conflict management skills through observation and participation (Hersh, 2008). For example, tested in the CPIC (Grych et al., 1992) was whether parents resolved their verbal conflict within time. This would indicate the possibility of learning conflict resolution strategies.

The study further identified other aspects children learned from their parents when in conflict. For example, verbal marital conflict exposed people within the family to anger and abuse, and this form of conflict opened opportunities for partners to be demeaning and psychologically abusive. Children exposed to this form of conflict learned the possibilities of valuing or devaluing others (Sturge-Apple, Skibi, & Davies, 2012). For example, during a conflict partners can call each other names that are demeaning which can teach their children such values. In other instances, partners may turn the child against the other partner during the conflict. Tested in this study with the CPIC (Grych et al., 1992) was if parents wanted a child to support or be on their side during a conflict.

The theoretical framework supporting the study was emotional security theory (EST) and social learning theory (SLT). EST recognized the potential for disagreements in relationship, and considered such a disagreement a problem if it caused violence, disengagement, and unresolved conversations (Davies & Cummings, 1994). This would then lead to doubt about a person's safety and the safety of other persons in the family. This study examined children's safety when their parents were in a verbal conflict. The results showed that children felt they were scared during the instances of conflict, where 26 participants indicating that this was *often always true*, and another 26 participants stating it was *often true,* and 21 participants stating it was *occasionally true*. The implications seemed to be verbal marital conflict was a cause for concern for children as it caused fear in the family. This aligns with EST. The family has an obligation to provide children with a sense of security (Davies & Cummings, 1994). Conflict denies them this feeling as it creates an atmosphere of disengagement and disregard for the well-being of others. The potential for causing emotional anxiety in children signifies that verbal conflict similar to other forms of conflict does affect the emotional security of children.

An aspect to note about EST is that children tend to feel safe or unsafe based on the level and type of conflicts they experience in the family (Davies & Cummings, 1994). They then form defense mechanisms based on the experiences. Emerging in this study was that sometimes when parents engaged in verbal conflict, children tried to intervene or do something to make themselves feel better. Children further formed defense mechanisms to use later when exposed to conflict such as becoming aggressive or detached. This study showed that participants did not have a challenge dealing with conflict as adults as they did not have an unmanageable temper or rash reactions. The study indicated that the responses of the participants was average even under provocation.

Underlying the second theory, SLT is the concept that the family is a socialization agent and children learn through the process of socialization in which they observe what others are doing rather than through coaching (Bandura, 1969). Based on SLT, children exposed to verbal marital conflict had a greater chance of developing skills used in such conflict compared to children that did not witness conflict. The skills gained could be positive or negative. For example, as tested here the children could learn conflict resolution skills if parents resolved their differences fast and amicably. The CPIC (Grych et al., 1992) tested if the participants felt their parents were able to resolve their differences, and a combined $n = 62$ chose the options of *occasionally true, often true,* and *often always true* signifying parents were able to identify solutions. Exposure to conflict management techniques could have a positive bearing on the way children would resolve their conflicts as adults. Although this was not part of the test for the current study, it is a premise that could develop based on the findings.

The current study provided an outlook on how adults exposed to verbal marital conflict as children formed anger reactions. The findings showed that exposure to verbal conflict did not mean a person would react angrily when confronted. Many of the participants indicated that their parents were able to resolve their conflicts, which could have had an implication on the participants. The study does not however look for that relationship. From the study, it emerges that the participants' responses were average, meaning that they do not show high tendencies to become angry or react in anger when confronted. However, many selected the position of *sometimes* when indicating whether they did react in anger or had a hot temper. A noted element was that the position of a considerable number of the participants felt they did not have anger challenges. Based on emotional responses the findings displayed average responses showing exposure to verbal marital conflict did not lead to poor anger responses in adulthood.

## Discussion of the Conclusions

The current study attempted to examine if there was a relationship between witnessing verbal marital conflict as a child and the behavior of anger responses as an adult. The findings showed there was no significant relationship between the feelings and responses of adults who experienced verbal conflicts between their parents as children and their anger in adulthood. This was a non-experimental correlation design comprised of surveys necessary to collect the data for the research. The criteria for the participants was to be 21 years of age and older, and to have witnessed verbal marital conflict as a child. The findings showed that a vast majority of the participants answered mid-level on the Likert type scales, which showed there was very little behavior anger responses by the participants.

**External Responses**

Previous research did not align with the findings in this study. Observation and participation are used by children to understand how to manage conflict within the family unit (Hersh, 2008). The literature showed that children exposed to parental verbal conflict may cause externalization and internalization of anger behaviors even as they grow into adulthood (El-Sheikh et al., 2009; Fosco & Grych, 2008; Obradovic, Bush, & Boyce, 2011). This information also explained why the slightest aggravation could cause a person to react violently as a way of defending oneself. In addition, literature found on externalization problems indicated children suffered from emotional challenges and self-blame (El-Sheikh et al., 2013; Zarling et al., 2013). The current study showed that children felt they were to blame for their parents' conflict with 27 participants selecting *often true*, and 47 participants selecting *almost always true*. Based on previous research detailing externalization problems, children who received poor socialization and poor conflict management would convey that same tactic to adulthood (Davies et al., 2012; Faircloth, 2012). This type of layover into adulthood provides an explanation as to why there are some people who have a difficult time preserving a decently cherished relationship. However, the current research displayed a dissimilar viewpoint. A vast amount of participants responded in the middle or low range of the Likert type scale in regards to reacting to anger responses. Many participants ($n = 81$) indicated they did not hit others, and 68 participants indicated that they did not slam things. However, when enquired if provoked they fly off the handle without knowing, 65 participants stated it was *not true*, 33 stated it was *sometimes true*, and two indicated it was *always true*.

Other characteristics children cultured from the conflicts of their parents was identified in this study as well. One example was exposure to verbal marital conflict within the family created an opening for other forms of conflict such as psychological abuse and humiliation. Children exposed to this form of conflict learned the possibilities of valuing or devaluing others (Sturge-Apple, Skibi, & Davies, 2012).

A challenge noted in the current study was that it was not easy to interpret the findings of the combined scales. The reason was that the scales were specific to the areas of their development. Individually, each scale provided critical insight into how children responded to exposure to marital conflict and the possible implications in adulthood. For example, the NAS (Novaco, 1994, 2003) showed a general outlook on how people responded when presented with conflicts. An example in the area of participants being rough with others where half of the participants ($n = 50$) indicated that sometimes they responded roughly; however, connecting this response to exposure to verbal conflict was difficult. This leads to a suggestion of conducting a qualitative study on the impact of verbal conflict on children. Despite the shortcoming, the study provided a good opportunity to assess how exposure to verbal marital conflict could influence adults. A majority of the participants were aged between 35 to 39 years with none being younger than 21 years of age.

**Aligned with EST**

The theoretical framework supporting the study was emotional security theory (EST) and social learning theory (SLT). Aligned with EST, the results from the study indicate 26% (*n* = 26) of participants responded with *often always true* when asked if they felt scared during the conflicts. There was a tie with 26 participants stating *often true* and 21 participants stating *occasionally true* in response to feeling scared during conflicts. Conflict denies children a sense of security (Davies & Cummings, 1994) and creates the possibility of children developing emotional anxiety. According to Davies and Cummings (1994), the level and forms of conflict children face assist them in how safe or unsafe they feel prior to forming defense mechanisms. Results of the current study showed that participants, when they were children, either tried to intervene or tried to do something to make themselves feel better; however, of those that tried to intervene 38 indicated *almost always true* in response to not being able to stop their parents from arguing. Additionally, 31 participants selected *occasionally true* in response to the statement regarding "...I could do something to make myself feel better..." when verbal marital conflict was present. Overall, based on the results of this study, it showed the responses to be average or under for adults showing no reactions of anger or recklessness due to witnessing marital conflict as a child.

**Aligned with SLT**

The second theory, Social Learning Theory (SLT), children learn through observing the socialization of the family (Bandura, 1969). Based on this theory, children who were exposed to verbal marital conflict produced a better chance of developing positive or negative skills used in the conflict. The current study tested through the CPIC (Grych et al., 1992) if participants felt their parents could resolve their differences. Sixty two of the participants felt this could be could be done and a resolution could be found. Seventy nine participants who experienced verbal marital conflict as a child selected *sometimes true* or *always true* in regards to yelling back in conflict. This could be explored in future research as a prevalent tool of awareness regarding conflict reaction. Children witnessing positive or negative conflict management techniques could have a bearing on how they resolve conflicts throughout their lives even to adulthood.

**Findings of the Current Study**

A viewpoint of anger response from adults who witnessed verbal marital conflict as children was delivered through the current study. The discovery disclosed that even though a person is exposed to verbal conflict, it did not indicate a person would react in an angered manner. Being that the participants scored high in their parents being able to resolve conflict (*almost always true* ($n = 14$), *often true* ($n = 24$), *occasionally true* ($n = 31$), *rarely true* ($n = 18$), and *almost never true* ($n = 13$)), this may have had an effect on the results; however, this information was not something the study was correlating. The overall results of the current study produced average responses showing there were no elevated characteristics of becoming angry even when confronted. Although many of the participants selected *sometimes true* they did react in anger for example, participants yelled back at people ($n = 68$) or responded roughly to people ($n = 50$), a vast number of participants felt they did not have anger issues who responded *never true* for instance, having a quick and hot temper ($n = 53$), flying off the handle ($n = 65$), taking out anger on others ($n = 78$) and knocking people around ($n = 77$). Based on the findings of the emotional responses and the mixed reactions in a few areas, witnessing verbal marital conflict as a child did not produce behavior anger responses in adulthood as shown by the average level of responses.

**Lack of Updated Research**

The last five years pertaining to published literature in this area is lacking. A review of SocIndex, PsycInfo, PsycArticles, ProQuest, SAGE Journals, Academic Search, and Goggle; exploring marital conflict and anger responses resulted with very little to no current research addressing the variables. In regards to the older literature in this area, anger response in association to verbal marital conflict does not provide a sufficient link between the two subjects in the current study. Therefore, after a thorough exploration, no updated research was found to support findings of the current study.

**Limitations**

This quantitative correlational study was limited in the use of the developed scales, understanding the use of wording, future risks, exploration of only verbal marital conflict, and the use of subscales. One limitation of this study was in the use of previously developed scales, which limited the researcher to focusing on the elements developed in these scales. This exposed the participants to a large number of questions that they did not need to answer for this study. The researcher could have also benefited from inclusion of some questions on perception, such as whether the conflict affected the child's performance in school and socially. It was suggested by Leedy and Ormrod (2005) that there is a limitation to accurately define constructs in survey research. Although the scales used asked the questions, their direct relationship to exposure to conflict was difficult to identify. Participants were limited to only the answers on the questionnaire and therefore could not express their feelings through expansion of their own words. A qualitative study could have addressed this issue, allowing participants to share their understanding of the paradigms presented (Creswell, 2007). Objective measures of the variables were explored through the use of quantitative measurement, whereas the subjective perception would have been defined using the qualitative measurement (Creswell, 2003). The study would benefit largely from a direct relationship. This does not however mean the questionnaire did not fulfill the research purpose as it did so within the identified limitation.

The study required the participants to have witnessed the verbal marital conflict. A limitation was found in the study concerning 24 participants who noted they almost never witnessed the verbal marital conflict. The response could be due to the participants misunderstanding the term "witnessing." The 24 participants who mentioned they almost never witnessed the verbal marital conflict may have felt that hearing the conflict and being in the same house, not necessarily in front to view the conflict was a way of witnessing it. Using a qualitative approach would have provided a more exploratory insight as to what the participant felt was the meaning to almost never witnessing the conflict. A self-administered questionnaire with space for the participant to expand on their experience would have been valuable (Finley, Baker, Pugh, & Peterson, 2010). As noted in the recommendation section below, it would be helpful in future research for the researcher to define the word "witness" as the researcher sees it fit to be used in the study.

Whether minimal or maximum, risks can be found in any study as no study is risk-free. Even though the researcher did not anticipate any participant would be harmed or distressed while participating in the study, there were some possible ways the participants could have experienced emotional risks such as: the participants could have questions for their parents about the reasons behind the conflicts and voice how it affected the participant's life, the participant could ask anyone living in the household such as a sibling; how did the conflicts affect them then and now, and the participant could have experienced emotional recollections of verbal marital conflicts. Although personal statements for further explanation were not allowed on the survey, having that personal touch would have added a bit of emotion to the study, which cannot be found in quantitative studies (Mertens, 2005). In the event the participant experienced any emotional risks, the consent form included a toll free counseling phone number for participants.

The study was limited to only verbal marital conflict situations. This provided a limited response to the questions on the survey. This also meant the participant needed to separate other acts of conflict to focus mainly on verbal marital conflict only. Even though these surveys have been used in previous similar research that does not erase the notion that participants could still apply subjectivity to the concept (Cochran & Fischer, 2007; Jonker, 2006; Navidian & Bahari, 2008). A definition for verbal marital conflict was provided to the participants in order for the respondents to provide the best possible answer pertaining to each marital conflict item on the questionnaire.

The NAS (Novaco, 1994, 2003) contains various subscales; however, only the behavior subscale was used for the results of this study. The behavior subscale served as a variable measuring the behavior anger responses of the adults during childhood. Using the entire NAS (Novaco, 1994, 2003) score could have provided a different marginal result for the study, but it would have also provided extended scale scores unnecessary to the desired variables of the study.

## Recommendations for Future Research or Interventions

The findings of this study pertain to those of adults exposed to verbal marital conflict as children. The gaps to the study; however, suggest the need for growing the study to include other elements. Therefore, suggestion for future study is to conduct a qualitative study examining the same phenomenon. The study would look at the effect of children witnessing verbal marital conflict with anger responses as adults. It may be beneficial to include the definition of "witness" in the context the researcher would like the participants to understand it in the study. According to Webster's dictionary (2014) the verb witness is defined as "to see something happen." Indicating exactly how the researcher perceives the word "witness" will have an effect on the data collection from the participants. The suggested data collection methods would be focus groups and interviews. The interviews would examine in depth the perceptions of adults who experienced verbal conflict as a child, while the focus group could serve a purpose of observation and reporting. The reporting would be participants indicating how exposure to parental conflict affected their response to anger provocation. Even though a survey could provide good results about people who witnessed parental conflict, it does not provide in depth information to promote a concrete conclusion on whether such exposure caused a poor reaction to anger response. Although this study recorded the demographics of ethnicity to demonstrate the diversity of those who participated; it was not, however, used as a variable in the research. For future research, it may be beneficial to research the role culture plays in how marital conflict is perceived, how different cultures manage marital conflict, and how children view the arguments in their cultured setting.

Another suggestion is to conduct a study examining how exposure to interparental conflict leads to certain behavior. Rather than using an established testing scale, the suggestion is to develop a new tool that would examine how participants reacted to stimulus. The study would identify quantitative measures. For example, the survey would ask participants whether they witnessed verbal marital conflict and request the participants to identify whether they could credit the experience with the way they reacted to situations. An example, the tool may ask whether the participants felt that exposure to verbal marital conflict led to their poor resolution of conflicts that occurred in their relationship. The suggestion is to have a clear connection in the study compared to the one found in the present study. Previous literature suggested that children's exposure to interparental conflict placed them at risk of developing maladjustment and behavioral problems (George, Davies, Cicchetti, & Sturge-Apple, 2013). Poor anger responses could be an example of maladjustment behaviors developing in children. However, children's behavior could differ depending on the age.

The counseling field can advance practice in addressing maladjustment in children exposed to parental conflict through person centered programs. These are programs that seek an understanding of the relationship between exposure to conflict, and patterns of response in the children such as stress activity. Based on the age of the child, the psychological adjustment will differ (Sturge-Apple, Skibi, & Davies, 2012). Through person-centered models, it would be possible to check for emotional insecurity, self-blame, and perceived threat experienced by children. The suggestion for person-centered intervention came from recognizing that children's reactions to parent conflict is not homogenous and therefore a homogenous approach to treatment could be inadequate

(Davies, Martin, & Cicchetti, 2012). Defining therapy based on the characteristics of the child, their reaction to conflict, and adjustment could offer a positive approach to treatment.

The current findings of this study have implications for policy development in family care. The suggestion is to enhance models of relationship skills training (Fomby & Osborne, 2007). Enhancement of how partners communicate is significant toward ensuring children will have a stable socialization environment. Families form the first contact the child has with conflict resolution (Driscoll & Nagel, 2011). For this reason, it will be important for families to have good communication mechanisms that children can emulate. The learned skills will have implications for the behavior children will adopt into adulthood. As the programs develop, they will need to consider working on improving the quality of relationships between couples and their interactions with the rest of the family. This should address the falsehood of considering that failing to show the conflict will not have an impact. Children are able to sense tension between their parents and can feel the conflict even though it remains hidden from them (Nicholas & Rasmussen, 2006). Another focus for family support groups is to help couples to limit the magnitude of children exposure to conflict between parents. Parents need to understand that they have a responsibility toward the development of their children and can have a positive impact if they provide quality conflict resolution skills. The goal of families or couples should not be hiding conflict from their children, but showing them that it is possible for people experiencing conflicts to arrive at an amicable solution.

The government has a role to play in policy development in ensuring adopted policies and programs are able to address the long and short-term influences of parental conflict on child development (Reynolds, 2014). Recognition of the role of such factors early in life is important in assisting counseling professionals and policy makers to identify and enhance positive results for children. This study and other studies noted in the literature review were able to show that children exposed to high intensity couple conflict could perpetuate the behaviors seen in their parents later (Ablow, Measelle, Cowan, & Cowan, 2009; Beuhler, et al., 2007; Davies & Cummings, 1998). The literature review also showed how children exposed to parental conflict are at risk of developing destructive resolutions; although they sometimes achieve constructive conflict resolution models (Strong et al., 2011). The adopted behavior has implications on how the children grow and whether they can achieve lasting relationships and deal with conflicts.

Another suggested program development could be in dialectical behavioral therapy (DBT) which could be useful in explaining the outcomes of experiencing verbal marital conflict as a child and behavior response in adulthood. Although this current study showed that a significant relationship did not exist between witnessing verbal marital conflict and anger response behavior as an adult, the DBT can guide further exploration of the issue. For example, some of the questions developed for the NAS (Novaco, 1994, 2003) and CPIC scales could act as a guideline for the aspects that a therapist would need to focus on. The use of the DBT would be in identifying persons who require therapeutic intervention following exposure to verbal marital conflict as children imparting on them skills to handle anger and violence. The DBT techniques would require a combination of behavioral science, dialectical philosophy of treatment, and Zen practices of acceptance and tolerance (Linehan, 1987, 1993; Miller et al., 2007;

Robins, 2000). It is suggested by Linehan (1987), a founder of DBT, that abusive behavioral problems are reflected through the client's skill deficit of emotion; therefore, a treatment plan will involve enhancing the emotional skill set of the client. In the case of this study, the behavioral problem would be verbal marital conflict. This type treatment plan can also be used to assist a client suffering from anger issues. The therapist should develop a comprehensive plan to include speaking openly about what was witnessed as a child, how it made the client feel then and now, how the client has coped with what was witnessed and when necessary have the client speak to others involved in the development of the anger issues, and use the empty chair technique when needed. These in-depth sessions could also include the involvement of the family in later sessions when the client seems ready and comfortable.

Therapists can also work with the client toward achieving healthy emotional, social, and interpersonal skills with the goal of helping the client form better future relationships. The findings of this study may act as a baseline for information on client exposure to verbal marital conflict and their reaction. Though the analysis provides a holistic outlook for all the participants, it can serve as an indicator for how children perceive verbal marital conflict, the behavior of parents during the conflict, and the development of children after the conflict. It offers a progressive outlook for children exposed to verbal marital conflict and their development into adulthood and anger responses.

## Conclusion

In conclusion, this study proved the null hypothesis meaning there was no significant relationship between witnessing verbal marital conflict as a child and anger responses in adulthood. The emerging correlation was 0.101 being greater than 0.05 which would have signified a relationship and proved the alternative hypothesis. However, noted in the study was that children reacted differently to their parents' arguments. For example, some of the participants indicated they felt they were to blame for their parents' arguments and sometimes tried to intervene. Another concern was that the children did feel that their parents sometimes wanted them to take sides. Despite such indications, the experiences did not mean the participant responded poorly to anger provocations in adulthood. The study noted that the participants sometimes reacted to provocation but many noted they did not have a hot temper. Therefore, experiencing verbal marital conflict as a child had no bearing on the response of the anger of the adult.

The findings of this study provide insight into how exposure to verbal marital conflict can influence some aspects of a child when growing up, although the significance in adult anger responses is lacking. This makes the study findings useful for therapeutic interventions for children exposed to verbal marital conflict as well as adults who failed to achieve healing from the exposure. For children, the findings indicate the anxiety that could develop, self-blame, and taking sides as shown on the CPIC (Grych et al., 1992). Therapists can use such findings as a guideline for their therapeutic sessions with children coming from homes with verbal marital conflict. The focus could be on: developing conflict resolution skills, helping the child understand their role in the family as a child rather than as the person to blame for the conflict, and working through their feelings related to the conflicts.

Based on the DBT, SLT, and EST; therapists can assist children and adults exposed to verbal marital conflict acquire the mental strength to overcome the negative implications of the conflict. SLT and EST offered in this study an element of understanding how conflicts occurring between a couple could affect the entire family, and affect the emotional development of their children. The theories can offer similar lessons during therapeutic intervention. The DBT would be the underlying intervention acting as a guide in development of appropriate action for persons exposed to verbal marital conflict.

# REFERENCES

Ablow, J. C., Measelle, J. R., Cowan, P. A., & Cowan, C. P. (2009). Linking marital conflict and children's adjustment: The role of young children's perceptions. *Journal of Family Psychology, 23*(4), 485-499. doi: 10.1037/a0015894

Adamson, J. L., & Thompson, R. A. (1998). Coping with interparental verbal conflict by children exposed to spouse abuse and children from nonviolent homes. *Journal of Family Violence, 13*(3), 213-232.

Amato, P. R. & Sobolewski, J. M. (2001). The effects of divorce and marital discord on adult children's psychological well-being. *American Sociological Review, 66*, 900-021.

Amedeo, D., Golledge, R. G., & Stimson, R. J. (2009). *Person-environment-behavior research: Investigating activities and experiences in spaces and environments.* New York, NY: The Guilford Press.

Akers, R. L., Krohn, M. D., Lanza Kaduce, L., & Radosevich, M. (1979). Social learning and deviant behavior: A specific test of general theory. *American Sociological Review, 44*(4), 636-655.

Baker, J. S., Fenning, R. M., & Crnic, K. A. (2011). Emotion socialization by mothers and fathers: Coherence among behaviors and associations with parental attitudes and children's social competence. *Social Development, 20*(2), 412-430.

Ballard, M. E., Cummings, E. M., & Larkin, K. (1993). Emotional and cardiovascular responses to adults' angry behavior and to challenging tasks in children of hypertensive and normotensive parents. *Child Development, 64*, 500–515.

Bandura, A. (1969). Social learning theory of identificatory processes. From D. A. Goslin (Ed), *Handbook of socialization theory and research* (pp. 213-262). Chicago: Rand McNally and Company.

Bandura, A. (1971). *Social learning theory.* Chicago: General Learning Corporation.

Bauer, N. S., Herrenkohl, T. I., Lozano, P., Rivara, F. P., Hill, K. G., & Hawkins, J. D. (2006). Childhood bullying involvement and exposure to intimate partner violence. *Pediatrics, 118*, e235–e242.

Berg, K. E., & Latin, R. W. (2008). *Essentials of research methods in health, physical education, exercise science, and recreation* (3$^{rd}$ ed.). Baltimore, MD: Lippincott Williams & Wilkins.

Berns, R. (2012). *Child, family, school, community: Socialization and support* (9th ed). Belmont, CA: Wadsworth, Cengage Learning.

Bickham N.L., & Fiese, B.H. (1997). Extension of the children's perceptions of interparental conflict scale for use with late adolescents. *Journal of Family Psychology, 11*, 246-250.

Bordens, K., & Abbott, B. (2011). *Research design and methods: A process approach* (8th ed). NY: McGraw Hill.

Bryman, A. (2012). *Social research methods* (4th ed). England: Oxford University Press.

Buehler, C. & Welsh, D. P. (2009). A process model of adolescents triangulation into parents marital conflict: The role of emotional reactivity. *Journal of Family Psychology, 23*(2), 167-180.

Buehler, C. (2014). *How marital conflict affects children.* The National Stepfamily Resource Center. Auburn, AL.

Bustillos-Perez, R. (2011). *Preventing relationship violence: Detection and intervention strategies for adolescents.* (Master's thesis). Available from ProQuest Dissertations and Theses database. (UMI No. 1508000)

Cannon, E. A., Bonomi, A. E., Anderson, M. L., Rivara, F. P., & Thompson, R. S. (2010). Adult health and relationship outcomes among women with abuse experiences during childhood. *Violence and Victims, 25*(3), 291-305. doi: 10.1891/0886-6708.25.3.291

Cavanagh, S. E., & Huston, A. C. (2006). Family instability and children's early problem behavior. *Social Forces, 85*, 551-581.

Cavanagh, S. E., Schiller, K. S., & Riegle-Crumb, C. (2006). Marital transitions, parenting, and schooling: Exploring the link between family-structure history and adolescents academic status. *Sociology of Education, 79*, 329-354.

Chow, S., Wang, H., & Shao, J. (2008). *Sample size calculations in clinical research* (2nd ed). Boca Raton, FL: Taylor and Francis Group.

Clarey, A., Hokoda, A., & Ulloa, E. C. (2010). Anger control and acceptance of violence as mediators in the relationship between exposure to interparental conflict and dating violence perpetration in Mexican adolescents. *Journal of Family Violence, 25*, 619-625. Doi: 10.1007/s10896-010-9315-7

Cooper, H. M. (1988). Organizing knowledge synthesis: A taxonomy of literature reviews. *Knowledge in Society, 1*, 104-126.

Corcoran, K., & Fischer, J. (2007). *Measures for clinical practice and research: A sourcebook* (4th ed.). New York, NY: Oxford.

Creswell, J.W. (2003). *Research design: Qualitative, quantitative, and mixed methods approaches* (2nd ed.). Thousand Oaks, CA: Sage.

Creswell, J.W. (2007). *Qualitative inquiry & research design: Choosing among five approaches* (2nd ed.). Thousand Oaks, CA: Sage.

Culhane, S. E. & Morera, O. F. (2010). Reliability and validity of the Novaco Anger Scale and Provocation Inventory (NAS-PI) and State-Trait Anger Expression Inventory-2 (STAXI-2) in Hispanic and non-Hispanic White student samples. *Hispanic Journal of Behavioral Sciences, 32*(4), 586-606.

Cummings, E. M. (1998). Children exposed to marital conflict and violence: Conceptual and theoretical directions. In G. W. Holden, R. Geffner, & E. N. Jouriles (Eds.), *Children exposed to marital violence: Theory, research, and applied issues* (pp. 55–93). Washington, DC: American Psychological Association.

Cummings, E. M., & Davies, P. T. (2002). Effects of marital conflict on children: Recent advances and emerging themes in process-oriented research. *Journal of Child Psychology and Psychiatry and Allied Disciplines, 43*, 31–63.

Cummings, E. M. & Davies, P. T. (2010). *Marital conflict and children: An emotional security perspective.* New York: The Guilford Press.

Cummings, E. M., Faircoth, W. B., Mitchell, P. M., Cummings, J. S., & Schermerhorn, A. C. (2008). Evaluating a brief prevention program for improving marital conflict in community families. *Journal of Family Psychology, 22*(2), 193-202.

Cummings, E. M., Kuoros, C. D., & Papp, L. M. (2007). Marital aggression and children's responses to everyday interparental conflict. *European Psychologist, 12*(1), 17-28.

Cummings, E. M., & Davies, P. (1996). Emotional security as a regulatory process in normal development and the development of psychopathology. *Development and Psychopathology, 8*, 123-139.

Davies, P. T., & Cummings, E. M. (2006). Interparental discord, family process, and developmental psychopathology. In D.Cicchetti & D. J.Cohen (Eds.), *Developmental psychopathology: Vol. 3. Risk, disorder, and adaptation* (2nd ed., pp. 86-128). NY: Wiley.

Davies, P. T., & Sturge-Apple, M. L. (2007). Advances in the formulation of emotional security theory: An ethologically based perspective. In R. V. Kail (Ed), *Advances in child development and behavior* (pp. 87-137). Elsevier.

Davies, P. T., & Woitach, M. J. (2008). Children's emotional security in the interparental relationship. *Current Directions in Psychological Science, 17*(4), 269-274. doi: 10.1111/j.1467-8721.2008.00588.x

Davies, P. T., Martin, M. J., & Cicchetti, D. (2012). Delineating the sequelae of destructive and constructive interparental conflict for children within an evolutionary framework. *Developmental Psychology, 48*(4), 939-95.

Davies, P.T., & Woitach, M.J. (2008). Children's emotional security in the interparental relationship. *Current Directions in Psychological Science*, 17, 269-274.

Davis, G. (2010). *Straight talk about communication research methods* (1$^{st}$ ed.). Iowa: Kendall Hunt Publishing Co. doi: 978-0-7575-7219-7

Dejonghe, E. S., Bogat, G. A., Levendosky, A. A., von Eye, A., & Davidson II, W. S. (2005). Infant exposure to domestic violence predicts heightened sensitivity to adult verbal conflict. *Infant Mental Health Journal, 26*(3), 268-281. doi: 10.1002/imhj.20048

Derscheid, L. & Allen, S. C. (2010). Quality of adult children's intimate relationships based on parental marital status and interparental conflict during children. Northern Illinois University, Consumer and Nutritional Sciences.

Driscoll, A., & Nagel, N. G. (2011). *Family socialization.* CA: Pearson Allyn Bacon Prentice Hall.

Edleson, J., & Nissley, B. (2011). *Emerging responses to children exposed to domestic violence.* National Resource Center on Domestic Violence. Retrieved from http://www.vawnet.org/applied-research-papers/print-document.php?doc_id=585

Elliott, D. B., & Simmons, T. (2011). Marital events of Americans: 2009. *American Community Survey Reports.*

El-Sheikh, M., Keiley, M., Erath, S., & Justin, D. W. (2013). Marital conflict and growth in children's internalizing symptoms: The role of autonomic nervous system activity. *Developmental Psychology, 49*(1), 92-108.

El-Sheikh, M., Kouros, C. D., Cummings, E. M., Keller, P., & Staton, L. (2009). Marital conflict and children's externalizing behavior: Pathways involving interactions between parasympathetic and sympathetic nervous system activity. *Monographs of the Society for Research in Child Development, 79*(1), vii-79.

Faircloth, B. (2012). Children and marital conflict: A review. *FIPP Casemakers, 6*(1), 1-5.

Fear, J. M., Champion, J. E., Reeslund, K. L., Forehand, R., Colletti, C., Roberts, L., & Compass, B.E. (2009). Parental depression and interparental conflict: Children and adolescents self-blame and coping responses. *Journal of Family Psychology, 23*(5), 762-766. doi: 10.1037/a0016381

Feldman, R., Mashalha, S., & Derdikman-Eiron, R. (2010). Conflict resolution in the parent-child, marital, and peer contexts and children's aggression in the peer group: A process-oriented cultural perspective. *Developmental Psychology, 46*(2), 310-325.

Finley, E. P., Baker, M., Pugh, M., & Peterson, A. (2010). Patterns and perceptions of intimate partner violence committed by returning veterans with post-traumatic stress disorder. *Journal of Family Violence, 25,* 737– 743. doi: 10.1007/s10896-010-9331-7

Fisher, S. D. (2012). *Mediators of interparental conflict and adolescent internalizing/externalizing behaviors.* (Doctoral dissertation). Retrieved from http://ir.uiowa.edu/cgi/viewcontent.cgi?article=3294&context=etd

Fomby, P. & Osborne, C. (2008). The relative effects of family instability and mother/partner conflict on children's externalizing behavior. *Presented in Session 110 of Family Structure Transitions and Child Well-Being.*

Fomby, P., & Cherlin. A. J. (2007). Family instability and child well-being. *American Sociological Review, 72,* 181-204.

Fosco, G. M., & Grych, J. H. (2008).Emotional, cognitive, and family systems mediators of children's adjustments to interparental conflict. *Journal of Family Psychology, 22*(6), 843-854.

Fosco, G. M., DeBoard, R. L., & Grych, J. H. (2007). Making sense of family violence: Implications of children's appraisals of interparental aggression for their short- and long-term functioning. *European Psychologist, 12*(1), 6-16.

Grusec, J. E. (2011). Socialization processes in the family: Social and emotional development. *Annual Review of Psychology, 62,* 243-269.

Grych, J. H., & Fincham, F. D. (1990). Marital conflict and children's adjustment: A cognitive-contextual framework. *Psychological Bulletin, 108*(2), 267-290. doi: 0033-2909/90/$00.75

Grych, J. H., Seid, M., & Fincham, F. D. (1992). Assessing marital conflict from the child's perspective: The children's perspective of interparental conflict scale. *Child Development, 63*(3), 558-572.

Grych, J., Oxtoby, C., & Lynn, M. (2013). The effects of interparental conflict on children. In M. A. Fine and F. D. Fincham (eds), *Handbook of family theories: A content based approach* (pp. 245-273). London: Routledge.

Hare, A. L., Miga, E. M., & Allen, J. P. (2008). Intergenerational transmission of aggression in romantic relationships: The moderating role of attachment security. *Journal of Family Psychology, 23*(6),808-818.

Heard, H. E. (2007a). The family structure trajectory and adolescent school performance. *Journal of Family Issues, 28*, 319-354.

Heard, H. E. (2007b). Fathers, mothers, and family structure: Family trajectories, parent gender, and adolescent schooling. *Journal of Marriage and Family, 69*, 435-450.

Heaton, T. B., & Forste, R. (2007). Informal unions in Mexico and the United States. *Journal of Comparative Family Studied, 38*, 55-69.

Hersh, M. (2008). *The impact of observed parental emotion socialization on adolescent self-medication* (Dissertation). Available from ProQuest Dissertations and Theses database. (UMI No. 3304273)

Heuristic. (2014). In *Merriam-Webster's online dictionary*. Retrieved from http://www.merriam-webster.com/dictionary/witness

Hornsveld, R. H., Muris, P., & Kraaimaat, F. W. (2011). The Novaco anger scale-provocation inventory (1994 version) in Dutch forensic psychiatric patients. *Psychological Assessment 23*(4), 937-944.

Howard, E. (2010). Using a free online questionnaire to determine the skills, competencies and knowledge required to work in a digital library environment in Australia. In A. Katsirikou & C. H. Skiadas (eds), Qualitative and quantitative methods in libraries: Theory and applications. *Proceedings of the International Conference on QQML2009.* London: World Scientific Publishing Co. Pte. Ltd.

Howden, L. M., & Meyer, J. A. (2011). Age and sex composition: 2010. *2010 Census Briefs.*

Jones, J., Thomas-Peter, B., & Gangstad, B. (2003). An investigation of the factor structure of the Novaco anger scale. *Behavioral and Cognitive Psychotherapy, 31*(4), 429-437.

Jonker, L. (2006). *Resilience factors in families living with a member with a mental disorder.* Published master's thesis, University of Stellenbosch, Matieland, Stellenbosch, South Africa.

Kassinove, H. (2014). *How to recognize and deal with anger.* Washington, D.C.: American Psychological Association.

Keller, P. S., Cummings, M., Davies, P. T., & Lubke, G. (2007). Children's behavioral reactions to marital conflict as a function of parents' conflict behaviors and alcohol problems. *European Journal of Developmental Psychology, 4*(2), 157-177.

Kerley, K. R., Xu, X., Sirisunyaluck, B., & Alley, J. M. (2010). Exposure to family violence in childhood and intimate partner perpetration or victimization in adulthood: Exploring intergenerational transmission in urban Thailand. *Journal of Family Violence, 25,* 337-347. doi: 10.1007/s10896-009-9295-7

Koss, K. J., George, M. R., Bergman, K. N., Cummings, E. M., Davies P. T., & Cicchetti, D. (2012). Understanding children's emotional processes and behavioral strategies in the context of marital conflict. *Journal of Child Psychology, 109*(3), 336-352.

Koss, K. L., George, M. R. W., Davies, P. T., Cicchetti, D., Cummings, E. M., & Sturge-Apple, M. L. (2013). Patterns of children's adrenocortical reactivity to interparental conflict and associations with child adjustment: A growth mixture modeling approach. *Development Psychology 49*(2), 317-26. doi: 10.1037/a0028246

Kuoros, C. D., Merrilees, C. E., & Cummings, M. (2008). Marital conflict and children's emotional security in the context of parental depression. *Journal of Marriage and the Family, 70*(3), 684-697.

Laurent, H. K., Kim, H. K., & Capaldi, D. M. (2008). Prospective effects of interparental conflict on child attachment security and the moderating role of parents' romantic attachment. *Journal of Family Psychology, 22*(3), 377-388.

Leedy, P. D., & Ormrod, J. E. (2005). *Practical research: Planning and design* (8th ed.). Upper Saddle River, NJ: Pearson Prentice Hall.

Leedy, P. D., & Ormrod, J. E. (2010). *Practical research: Planning and design* (9$^{th}$ ed.). Upper Saddle River, NJ: Pearson Education, Inc.

Lindahl, K. M. & Malik, N. M. (2011). Marital conflict typology and children's appraisals: The moderating role of family cohesion. *Journal of Family Psychology, 25*(2), 194-201.

Linehan, M.M. (1987). Dialectical behavioral therapy: A cognitive behavioral approach to parasuicide. *Journal of Personality Disorders, 1*(4), 328-333.

Linehan, M. M. (1993). *Cognitive-behavioral treatment of borderline personality disorder.* New York, NY: Guilford Press.

Lochman, J. E., Barry, T., Powell, N., & Young, L. (2010). Anger and aggression. In D. W. Nangle, D. J. Hansen, C. A. Erdley, & P. J. Norton (eds), *Practitioner's guide to empirically based measures of social skills* (pp. 118-142). New York: Springer.

Lumsden, J. (2007). Online questionnaire design guidelines. In R. A. Reynolds, R. Woods, and J. D. Baker, *Handbook of research on electronic survey and measurements* (pp. 420-439) . London: Idea Group.

Luster, T., & Okagaki, L. (2011). *Parenting: An ecological perspective.* London: Routledge.

Mertens, D.M. (2005). *Research and evaluation in education and psychology* (2nd ed.). Thousand Oaks, CA: Sage.

McIntosh, J. (2010). Children's response to separation and parental conflict. *Every Child Magazine, 16*(2), 1. Retrieved from http://www.earlychildhoodaustralia.org.au /every_child_magazine/every_child_index/childrens_responses_to_separation_an d_parental_conflict.html

Miller, A. L., Rathus, J. H., & Linehan, M. M. (2007). *Dialectical behavioral therapy with suicidal adolescents.* New York, NY: The Guilford Press.

Mirabile, S. P. (2010). *Emotion socialization, emotional competence, and social competence and maladjustment in early childhood.* (Doctoral dissertation). Retrieved from http://scholarworks.uno.edu/cgi/viewcontent.cgi?article= 2142&context=td

Moura, O., Santos, R. A., Rocha, M., & Mantos, P. M. (2010). *Children's perception of interparental conflict scale (CPIC): Factor structure and invariance across adolescents and emerging adults.* NY: Taylor and Francis.

Moura, O., Santos, R. A., Rocha, M., & Matos, P. M. (2010). Children's Perception of Interparental Conflict Scale (CPIC): Factor structure and invariance across adolescents and emerging adults. *International Journal of Testing, 10,* 364-382.

Myers, D. (1995). Eliminating the battering of women by men: Some considerations for behavioral analysis. *Journal of Applied Behavioral Analysis, 28,* 493-507.

Nauert, R. (2012). Marital Troubles May Have Long-Term Effect on Kids. *Psych Central*. Retrieved from http://psychcentral.com/news/2012/06/15/marital-troubles-may-have-long-term-effect-on-kids/40210.html

Navidian, A., & Bahari, F. (2008). Burden experienced by family caregivers of patients with mental disorders. *Pakistan Journal of Psychological Research, 23,* 19-28.

Nicholas, K. B., & Rasmussen, E. H. (2006). Childhood abusive and supportive experiences, inter-parental violence, and parental alcohol use: Symptoms and aggression. *Journal of Family Violence, 21*(1), 43-61. DOI: 10.1007/s10896-005-9001-3.

Nigg, J. T., Nikolas, M., Miller, T., Burt, S. A., Klump, K. L., et al. (2009). Factor structure of the children's perception of interparental conflict scale for studies of youths with externalizing behavior problems. *Psychological Assessment, 21*(3), 450-456.

Nikolas, M., Klump, K., Burt, S. (2012). Youth Appraisals of Inter-parental Conflict and Genetic and Environmental Contributions to Attention-Deficit Hyperactivity Disorder: Examination of GÃ—E Effects in a Twin Sample. *J Abnormal Child Psychology, 40*(4), 543-554. doi: 10.1007/s10802-011-9583-6

Novaco, R. W. (n.d.). *The Novaco anger scale and provocation inventory.* Manson Western Corporation.

Novaco, R.W. (2003). *Novaco anger scale and provocation inventory (NAS-PI).* Western Psychological Services, Los Angeles, CA.

Obradovic, J., Bush, N. R., Boyce, W. T. (2011). The interactive effect of marital conflict and stress reactivity on externalizing and internalizing symptoms: The role of laboratory stressors. *Developmental Psychopathology, 23*(1), 101-114.

Osborne, C. & McLanahan, S. (2007). Partnership instability and child well-being. *Journal of Marriage & Family, 69,* 1065-1083.

Pauli-Pott, U., & Beckermann, D. (2007). On the association of interparental conflict with developing behavioral inhibition and behavior problems in early childhood. *Journal of Family Psychology, 21*(3), 529-532.

Quarles, R. C. (2001). Blurring the traditional boundaries between qualitative and quantitative research. *CASRO*. Retrieved from http://www.qsaresearch.com/Blurring%20Differences.pdf

Randolph, J. J. (2009). A guide to writing the dissertation literature review. *Practical Assessment, Research & Evaluation, 14*(13), 1-13. Retrieved from http://pare online.net/getvn.asp?v=14&n=13

Reinecke, M. A., Dattilio, F. M., & Freeman, A. (2003). *Cognitive therapy with children and adolescents: A casebook for clinical practice.* New York, NY: The Guilford Press.

Rhoades, K. A. (2009). Children's responses to interparental conflict: A meta-analysis of their associations with child adjustment. *Child Development, 79*(6).

Richmond, M. K., & Stocker, C. M. (2007). Changes in children's appraisals of marital discord from childhood through adolescent. *Journal of Family Psychology, 21*(3): 416-425.

Robinson, J. H. (2009). *Interpersonal conflict and child adjustment: The role of child optimism.* (Doctoral dissertation). Retrieved from http://ir.uiowa.edu/etd/424/

Sween, M. (2011). *Marital conflict, negative temperament and problem behaviors of children: A test of stability and variability across time.* (Doctoral dissertation). Retrieved from http://lib.dr.iastate.edu/cgi/viewcontent.cgi?article=1022&context=etd

Shelton, K. H. & Harold, G. T. (2008). Pathways between interparental conflict and adolescent psychological adjustment. *Journal of Early Adolescence.* doi: 10.1177/0272431608317610

Siegel, L., & Welsh, B. (2009). *Juvenile delinquency: Theory, practice, and law.* Independence, KY: Cengage Learning.

Simon, V. A., & Furman, W. (2010). Interparental conflict and adolescents' romantic relationship conflict. *Journal of Research on Adolescence, 20*(1), 188-209. doi: 10.1111/j.1532-7795.2009.00635.x

Singh, G. (2010). *What the concept of emotional security means for children.* Denver, CO: Clarity Digital Group, LLC.

Strong, B., DeVault, C., & Cohen, T. F. (2011). *The marriage and family experience: Intimate relationship in a changing society* (11th ed.). Belmont, CA: Wadsworth Cengage Learning.

Sturge-Apple, M. L., Davies, P. T., Winter, M. A., Cummings, E. M., & Scermerhorn, A. (2008). Interparental conflict and children's school adjustment: The explanatory role of children's international representations of interparental and parent-child relationships. *Developmental Psychology, 44*(6), 1679-1690.

Sturge-Apple, M. L., Skibo, M. A., & Davies, P. T. (2012). Impact of parental conflict and emotional abuse on children and families. *Partner Abuse, 3*(3).

Tavistock Center for Couple Relationships, The. (2012). The impact of couple conflict on children. *Policy Briefing*. Retrieved from http://tccr.ac.uk/images/uploads/policy_use/policybriefings/TCCR_impact_of_couple_conflict_briefing.pdf

Tedwater, R. (2010). *Effects of marital conflict on children*. Mys Sahana. Retrieved from http://www.mysahana.org/2010/11/marital-conflict-children/

Towe-Goodman, N. R., Stifter, C. A., Coccia, M. A., Cox, M. J., & The Family Life Project Key Investigator. (2011). Interparental aggression, attention skills, and early childhood behavior problems. *Development and Psychopathology, 23*, 563-576. doi: 10.1017/S095457411000216

Turcotte-Seabury, C. A. (2010). Anger management and the process mediating the link between witnessing violence between parents and partner violence. *Violence and Victims, 25*(3), 306-318. doi: 10.1891/0886-6708.25.3.306

U.S. Census Bureau. (2012). *Statistical abstract of the United States: 2012*. Retrieved from http://quickfacts.census.gov/qfd/states/00000.html

Van Gelder, M. M., Bretveld, R. W., & Roeleveld, N. (2010). Web-based questionnaires: The future in epidemiology? *American Journal of Epidemiology, 172*(11), 1292-1298.

Walckner, S. (2011). *Long-term effects of conflict on children*. Marital Mediation. Retrieved from http://www.maritalmediation.com/2011/09/long-term-effects-of-conflict-on-children/

Wright, K. B. (2005). Research internet-based populations: Advantages and disadvantages of online survey research, online questionnaire authoring software packages, and web survey services. *Journal of Computer-Mediated Communication, 10*(3).

Wymbs, B. T. (2008). *Does disruptive child behavior cause interparental discord? An experimental manipulation*. Ann Arbor, MI: ProQuest LLC.

Yip, V., Gudijonsson, G., Perkins, D., Doidge, A., Hopkin, G, Young, S. (2013). A non-randomised controlled trial of the R&R2MHP cognitive skills program in high risk male offenders with severe mental illness. *BMC Psychiatry, 13*, 267. doi: 10.1186/1471-244X-13-267.

Zarling, A. L., Taber-Thomas, S., Murray, A., Knuston, J. F., & Lawrence, E. (2013). Internalizing and externalizing symptoms in young children exposed to intimate partner violence: Examining intervening processes. *Journal of Family Psychology, 27*(6), 945-955.

Zeanah, C. H. (2012). *Handbook of infant mental health* (3rd ed). New York, NY: Guilford Press.

www.ingramcontent.com/pod-product-compliance
Lightning Source LLC
Chambersburg PA
CBHW070953080526
44587CB00015B/2287